Perinatal Loss

A HANDBOOK FOR WORKING WITH WOMEN AND THEIR FAMILIES

SHEILA BRODERICK
CQSW, Dip. SW
Senior Women's Health Counsellor

and

RUTH COCHRANE
MD, FRCOG
Consultant Obstetrician and Gynaecologist

Foreword by
JULIA GRAY
Chair, South East London Sands
(Stillbirth & Neonatal Death Society)

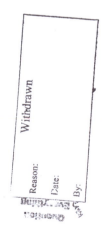

Radcliffe Publishing
London • New York

Radcliffe Publishing Ltd
33–41 Dallington Street
London
EC1V 0BB
United Kingdom

www.radcliffehealth.com

British Library Cataloguing in Publication Data

A catalogue record for this book is available from the British Library.

ISBN-13: 978 184619 980 6

The paper used for the text pages of this book is FSC® certified. FSC (The Forest Stewardship Council®) is an international network to promote responsible management of the world's forests.

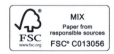

MIX
Paper from
responsible sources
FSC® C013056

Typeset by Darkriver Design, Auckland, New Zealand
Printed and bound by TJI Digital, Padstow, Cornwall, UK

Contents

Foreword

This is an important and warmly welcomed book which thoroughly endorses the key aims of Sands (Stillbirth & Neonatal Death Society). In particular, it demonstrates a forceful commitment to improving care for bereaved families whilst acknowledging the difficult task that staff undertake when caring for them. This handbook encompasses all aspects of perinatal loss, giving due care and attention to the many different circumstances and exploring the thoughts and feelings which are experienced when a baby dies at any gestation.

My daughter Grace was stillborn in September 1996 at 39 weeks in a large London teaching hospital. My community midwife had called on me at home and was unable to find a heartbeat. I was aware that I hadn't felt her move for a few days but, like so many women I have met through Sands, didn't think for a minute that she might be stillborn. What possible cause was there for a healthy full term baby to die? It was this ignorance, coupled with fear, that accompanied me to hospital on that Thursday in September. I desperately wanted to know what might have happened and what was going to happen. How was I going to cope? Giving birth to death is contrary to nature. My partner joined me for the night, and my midwife began the process of induction. It was the loneliest, most frightening night of my life. I felt totally unprepared for the ordeal and once my midwife had gone home, asking to be paged when labour was established, I was effectively 'abandoned'. Staffing levels were blamed for the fact that I had no professional care for the entire night or most of the following morning. At the moment of my daughter's head crowning, my partner was screaming for help down the corridor. My midwife arrived after Grace was born and had not been paged, as requested. The essential qualities referred to in this handbook on page 48 – compassion, empathy and responsiveness to needs – were signally absent in my case, and compounded my awful sense of failure, isolation and unworthiness. I wish I had received the care which I know is becoming more widely practised and could reflect on the tragedy without anger and hurt but with the knowledge that my daughter's life was demonstrably respected and validated through the sensitive communication of the staff.

It is heartening to know that two highly respected health professionals, Sheila Broderick and Ruth Cochrane, have dedicated their time and energy to writing this book. They have many years of experience and have evidently listened to bereaved parents and staff, not only exploring the highly complex feelings and emotions which have arisen in their practice, but also recognising the importance of the management of the practical aspects of the care. I am struck by one of the significant and recurring themes in this book and that is: 'each and every loss is individual to the patient involved'. My work with Sands brings me into contact with women and their partners, all with their own unique experiences and strategies for living with the reality of this life-changing event. This book can only enhance the work we do and will prove an invaluable resource. I feel privileged to have been invited to contribute and will continue to promote the highest standards of care which I know play such a significant part in the grieving process.

Julia Gray
Chair, South East London Sands
(Stillbirth & Neonatal Death Society)
October 2012

About the authors

Sheila Broderick is Senior Women's Health Counsellor at University Hospital Lewisham. She has worked there for 15 years, offering a direct service to bereaved women and their families, as well as working with her colleagues in a multi-disciplinary team to improve services for patients who suffer a pregnancy loss. Before becoming a counsellor, Sheila worked in the voluntary sector following her initial training as a social worker. She has worked with people with mental health problems, in a therapeutic drug rehabilitation centre and offers teaching and training in adult education.

Ruth Cochrane is Consultant Obstetrician and Gynaecologist at University Hospital Lewisham. She has been a consultant since 1997 and is a busy generalist with interests in high-risk obstetrics, major benign gynaecological surgery and undergraduate education. She became a Fellow of the Royal College of Obstetricians and Gynaecologists in 2003. Ruth developed an interest in the management of perinatal loss while she was a registrar, undertaking specialist training at the Tavistock Centre and supported ever since by her midwifery colleagues.

Abbreviations

ACA	anti-cardiolipin antibody
APS	anti-phospholipid syndrome
ARC	Antenatal Results and Choices
CHI	chronic histiocytic intervillositis
CS	caesarean section
CTG	cardiotocograph
CVS	chorionic villus sampling
DCDA	dichorionic diamniotic
D&E	dilatation and evacuation
EDD	expected date of delivery
EPAU	early pregnancy assessment unit
ERPC	evacuation of retained products of conception
FSE	fetal scalp electrode
GA	general anaesthetic
GP	general practitioner
HTA	Human Tissue Authority
IUFD	intrauterine fetal death
IVF	in vitro fertilisation
MCDA	monochorionic diamniotic
MCMA	monochorionic monoamniotic
MDU	Medical Defence Union
MPS	Medical Protection Society
NMC	Nursing and Midwifery Council
PCA	patient-controlled analgesia
PM	post-mortem
Sands	Stillbirth & Neonatal Death Society
TOP	termination of pregnancy
TTTS	twin-to-twin transfusion syndrome
UK	United Kingdom
VBAC	vaginal birth after caesarean

CHAPTER 1

Introduction

The aim of this book is to shed some light on the issues for all those involved in caring for patients who experience a pregnancy loss. The end of a pregnancy, at whatever gestation, can be both physically frightening and emotionally painful and being looked after by professionals who care can make an otherwise unbearable experience bearable. More than anything, we want those looking after a mother and father whose baby dies to have a sense of pride and honour in relation to the care they provide.

The experience of a couple whose baby dies and who feel cared for by staff is hugely different from that of a couple who have a similar loss but do not feel cared for. The first will say that the staff 'did everything they could' and were wonderful and caring, and that they almost had a positive experience in the midst of their grief. The second will have noticed every little thing that was not done correctly or every phrase said to them that was insensitive, and may even attribute the death of their baby to the lack of care they received. This can happen prior to the death of the baby: for example, a woman who was worried about her baby but was refused a scan without adequate explanation may think that if she had been given a scan any problems would have been identified and acted upon. It can also happen at the time of giving birth: a woman may remember a delay in being taken to theatre for a trial of instrumental delivery and think that without the delay the baby may have survived. In the course of our work with bereaved couples, we have often been told 'if only we had been cared for differently, perhaps our baby would have lived'. Occasionally, this will actually be true, but when it is not, it is very hard for couples to believe that this is the case. Lack of fundamental care can make parents suspicious of the motives of all caregivers and they will distrust feedback that can, to them, sound like a cover-up.

To highlight some of these issues, we have given examples throughout the book of both good and bad care. We hope that by discussing patients' bad experiences, you will learn from these and therefore be more confident when dealing with bereaved parents in the future.

There is a collective myth, at least in this society, that getting pregnant, staying pregnant, giving birth to a live baby and having a baby that survives is simple, despite clear evidence that this is not the case. There is an assumption that it is easy and within people's control. A woman who uses an ovulation predictor kit and gets pregnant soon afterwards will attribute her pregnancy to using the kit and feel that she had control over her conception, whereas our experience tells us that she was simply fortunate to get pregnant that month. Women who use predictor kits and never get pregnant can attest to this. It is partly this myth that women are up against when they experience a pregnancy loss. If a woman believes that her pregnancy will be normal and result in a healthy baby, she is protecting herself from the notion that something will go wrong. Women also think that things can go wrong with other people's pregnancies but not their own. They believe that all will be well once they are pregnant and that their baby will be born alive and will thrive. Why else would women who are only 12 weeks pregnant start decorating the nursery and buying baby clothes? We, the caregivers, need to understand this myth so that we can recognise the myriad reactions women and their families have in response to a pregnancy loss. For example, women who have experienced a baby dying will mention that they feel like outsiders and that other people have what they have not. It will seem to them that babies and pregnant women are everywhere. They are often very aware of how children are being treated and if they are not being treated well this exacerbates their feeling of 'Why me?' and their sense of unfairness. They are no longer able to buy into the collective myth that all will be well.

We work in a diverse multicultural borough in London and are aware of the varied ways that people from different cultures cope with pregnancy loss. However, we have deliberately not made significant reference to these differences in our book, as we are wary of making distinctions that do not account for individuals within any particular culture. We want people to be treated as individuals and not grouped together by what is defined as their 'culture'. Not all members of a perceived culture will react in the same way. For example, we once heard it said 'African women do not want to see or hold their babies' only to have this contradicted by an African midwife whose own baby had died. Cultural norms are collective; thus, to apply blanket beliefs to

individuals is likely to do as much harm as being completely ignorant of them. Furthermore, until relatively recently, it was the cultural norm in Britain that newly bereaved mothers be separated from their dead babies immediately. It was thought that it was better for and kinder to women and their families to relieve them of the burden of seeing, holding or taking any responsibility for their babies. Nowadays, we see the error of this reasoning and know how in the past it harmed women, who then spent a lifetime wondering what happened to their son or daughter.

Our book covers both the practical and emotional aspects of caring for bereaved parents and their families. The focus is principally on the mother, but we have tried to acknowledge the significance of the loss for her partner and her extended family where it is appropriate.

There are some over-arching principles that cover all aspects of pregnancy loss that we discuss below.

COMMUNICATION

Good communication is at the heart of this work and is one of the ways in which people know they are cared for. Communication is a two-way process: it includes the way someone is spoken to – what is said or not said – as well as what is understood. It is complex and there needs to be an appreciation of the patient's position before it can be said to be occurring. Patients come to hospital with many assumptions about the role of the doctor, nurse or midwife. Most patients will expect to be looked after. They can be in awe of you and expect you to be an expert. They can be worried about taking up too much of your time and scared of being thought wrong or stupid. They may attempt to communicate but give up because they are not being heard. These concerns are unlikely to be voiced, but they will manifest themselves in the way that the patient behaves: some will be aggressive and others will be passive. Aggressive patients are difficult to deal with, but it is important to see beyond their aggression, as they are likely to be worried and will use anger or hostility to hide this. Passive patients will not cause any trouble and it may be easy not to notice their concerns, but it is vital that you do.

Communication requires time. This can be difficult, but it behoves you to ensure that both the patient and yourself have enough time to enable it to happen. It may mean risking annoying colleagues by concentrating on one patient and leaving them to deal with the others. Fear of getting it wrong can interfere with the ability to communicate or making the time and effort required to stay with a distressed mother. There will be practical tasks that are the same for each pregnancy loss and the emotional response may be similar, but how both the tasks and the communication are undertaken will vary according to the patient you are dealing with each time.

PATIENT-CENTRED CARE

'Patient-centred care' means putting patients at the heart of their treatment. It means taking your cues from the patient and using active listening skills. Active listening skills are part of good communication. Worries need to be taken seriously and then if they are found to be groundless, so much the better, and you will have a patient who feels respected and acknowledged. Women report that they have sensed that something was wrong with their baby and been worried, only to be told by a doctor or midwife not to worry. It is important to know that if they had any choice about not worrying, then they would not worry. To say to someone 'don't worry' is at best dismissive; at worst, if their worries prove to be correct, the patient will be left feeling hurt, frustrated and powerless. She will say 'if only they had listened' and think that it might have made a difference if they had done so.

No matter how many pregnancy-loss cases you have managed, you need to know that each and every loss is individual to the patient involved. The end of a pregnancy may be the patient's first experience of a difficulty in pregnancy or she may have previously had a loss or losses. You need to take your cues from her as to how she wants to be treated. You may need to tell her what her options are, give her support whilst she decides which of these to choose and help her by making any necessary arrangements. It may be that patients make choices that surprise or unsettle you. An example of this would be a woman choosing to continue a pregnancy when the baby has been diagnosed with a lethal congenital abnormality. You need to be able to listen and be supportive, rather than voice any confusion or disapproval. Neither should you tell the woman what you would do in the same circumstances. It is her pregnancy and her decision, and you must show her that you support her, whatever she decides.

Another example of taking your cue from the patient is when you are referring to the baby's sex. Some couples will not want to know the sex of their stillborn baby, which may be a defence mechanism – if they do not know whether their baby was a boy or a girl, they cannot get too close, or so they believe. For others, knowing the baby's sex is intrinsic to their grieving process. They can refer to losing their daughter or their son and using these words helps them to start to make sense of their loss.

TRY NOT TO MAKE ASSUMPTIONS

Both patients and staff will make assumptions about pregnancy loss. Patients make assumptions about why the pregnancy went wrong in an effort to make sense of their loss, and staff make assumptions because it feels better to discuss a reason for the death than to admit that you do not know why it happened. Both of these reactions are strategies for managing the situation, but it can be very hard to unravel any misunderstandings if the original assumption was incorrect. Therefore, we would say that unfortunately there are no rules to follow other than never to make assumptions. If there were rules, then it would make the profound task of looking after a woman when her baby dies that much simpler.

The majority of people will want to know why this tragedy has happened to them. They will search for answers: they may scour the Internet and will review what they did or did not do that might have caused the loss; they will remember the glass of wine they drank or the heavy box they lifted. You may be tempted to respond to their questions, but do not guess if you do not know the answer; it is distressing to the patient to be told something that they later find out to be incorrect.

You may want to tell people what you think has happened because they ask you. You may find yourself saying things like 'you'll need a stitch next time' or 'the cord was wrapped around the baby's neck', but you need to resist answering any questions until such time as any cause of death has been established.

USE OF APPROPRIATE LANGUAGE

In writing this book, we have realised that the issue of the use of appropriate language comes up in several different ways. There is our use of language in this book, which we will discuss further in a moment; there is patients' use of language and how that can differ from the way that staff speak; there is the risk of causing upset or offence to patients if we use language insensitively.

Even though this is primarily a book for staff rather than patients, we have made a deliberate effort to use language in a personal rather than clinical way. Doctors in particular may distance themselves from their patients' agony by talking about what is going on in a detached and impersonal manner. As a contrast, we have used words that patients rather than doctors would use and tried to avoid euphemisms or any words that hide or belittle the truth. So, for example, we say 'their baby' rather than 'the baby', and try to say 'death' rather than 'loss'. We have also used 'he' or 'she' rather than 'it' when referring to babies, swapping between sexes throughout each chapter.

Patients' use of language is often very different from that of medical staff. We should do our best to use the same words as the patients. As an example, we have used the word 'baby' throughout the book, except when talking about the first trimester, when we have used the word 'fetus'. We have done this deliberately because it reflects the way that some women will use the word 'fetus' early on, until the pregnancy is more established. Some will not say 'baby' for fear of becoming attached to a pregnancy that they might lose, or they may feel that it is not a baby until a certain gestation. Others will say 'baby' from the beginning, which can be unnerving for some staff, especially in the context of a pregnancy going wrong in the first few weeks. We do not make a distinction between the relative importance of the two words 'baby' and 'fetus', and when working with a woman we would use the word 'baby' from the start if this is what she uses.

We have referred to couples sometimes as being a mother and her partner and sometimes as a mother and father. We are aware that same-sex couples and women without a partner, either by choice or not, have pregnancy losses, but we have not made these distinctions in the book for ease of writing.

RECOGNISING THE CHALLENGES

It is very important that, in the face of something awful happening, you do not become paralysed. We need to be aware of our own attitudes towards pregnancy loss, which aspects of a baby dying we find easier or harder to deal with and why that is. We need to strive to get it right, but it is important to be aware that it may not be possible to get it right for every patient every time. This is because each patient, her partner and her family are unique and will react to what has happened in their own individual ways. One example of this is in telling someone that you are scanning that they have suffered an intrauterine death. You may try to be kind by being indirect – 'I can see the chambers of the heart here, and as you can see they are not moving, and I'm afraid this means that your baby's heart is not beating, and so . . .' – but some patients would prefer you to come straight out with it: 'I am sorry to say that your baby has died'. Others would construe this as being too blunt. You may find that you are criticised whatever you do; you have to learn that this is part of the complexity of a baby dying and not blame the patient for her reaction to the dreadful news of her baby's death.

We tend to live in a culture of blame: it is common to see advertisements that encourage insurance claims when accidents have happened. We believe there is a huge difference between blaming individuals and people taking

responsibility for their mistakes. Mistakes are opportunities for learning and in the health profession there are sometimes near misses and sometimes dire consequences of mistakes. We want to emphasise that the hospital in which the two of us work is no different from any other in this regard: despite the best care, some pregnancies go wrong and usually no one is to blame. However, it is crucial that the organisation and individuals within it take responsibility for any mistakes that surround the death of a baby, including errors that might have contributed to the baby dying. Patients find it much easier to handle dreadful blunders if, from the outset, there is no attempt to cover them up. We would add that it is vital that the patient's experience of what happened forms a key part of any investigation, as their experience can differ greatly from that of the others involved. From the outset, the investigating team should not take an adversarial approach. This does not mean that patients are exclusively correct; rather, it means that their experiences need to be appreciated, as you cannot disagree with or dispute someone else's experience. In an atmosphere where blame is not the first resort, staff will feel safe enough to talk about their experience and be able to explain their decision-making.

Finally, in most cases in which a pregnancy loss is beyond anyone's control, you need to know that whilst you cannot change anything or put it right, you can do something very meaningful. Do what you can to make the patient's experience the best it can be and get help to do the things that you cannot. This maxim is a broad one, as it can mean asking a senior colleague to help manage an unfamiliar case or acknowledging that another member of the team may be better placed than you to help the patient. You cannot always get it right, but you can learn to live with this fact if your intentions towards the patient are good and you do your best to be kind and professional. We realise how hard this can be and that is why we have written this book.

CHAPTER 2

Types of losses

INTRODUCTION

This chapter discusses the different types of pregnancy loss and illustrates some of the emotional impact that these losses can have for women and their families.

USE OF LANGUAGE: WHY DEFINITIONS CAN BE PROBLEMATIC

We think it is worth starting this chapter with a discussion of the use of language in relation to pregnancy loss. Language is very important in this context because the use of insensitive language can be unexpectedly hurtful. For example, we are aware that as we write, members of the Miscarriage Association are trying to find different terminology for the evacuation of retained products of conception (ERPC), as women have told them that it is confusing and distressing to have the end of their pregnancy described this way.

Strictly speaking, in medical terminology, the word 'miscarriage' means 'the loss of a pregnancy before 24 completed weeks'. Most miscarriages occur in the first trimester, so for most women 'miscarriage' means the loss of a pregnancy in the first 3 months. The *Oxford English Dictionary* defines miscarriage as 'the spontaneous or unplanned expulsion of a fetus from the womb before it is able to survive independently'.[1] This is slightly different from the medical definition and does not specify a gestation. It highlights the distinction that most non-medical people would understand about the difference between a fetus (that could not survive outside its mother) and a baby (that could survive outside its mother and for whom the word 'miscarriage' would not be appropriate).

The *Collins Thesaurus* lists several synonyms for 'miscarriage' that make it clear that the word means something has gone very wrong and/or that a mistake has been made.[2] These synonyms include 'botch', 'error', 'mishap', 'failure' and 'perversion'. In another use of the word, the term 'miscarriage of justice' is defined as 'a failure of a court or judicial system to attain the ends of justice, especially one which results in the conviction of an innocent person'.[1] The English language makes it clear that 'miscarriage' means 'failure', and although as doctors and midwives we may believe that we are talking about a failure of nature, it is easy to understand why women who miscarry feel that it is their bodies that have failed or that they themselves have failed.

Some women will talk about miscarriage in terms of failure rather than of nature, or a failure not of that particular pregnancy but of themselves: 'I lost the baby', not 'our baby was lost'. They will talk about what happened in language that makes it clear that they perceive that the loss was in some way their fault: 'my cervix was too weak to hold on to the pregnancy'; 'I tried to do everything right but it wasn't enough'. Even though the pregnancy loss is clearly not her fault, this does not stop a woman from believing that this is the case and metaphorically beating herself up. This is especially the case if there is anything in her history that she may attribute to causing the miscarriage: 'I had a termination when I was 15'. In this way, women can characterise a miscarriage as some form of divine justice or karma because of something that happened years ago that has now come back to haunt them. Whatever the rights and wrongs of this analysis (and it may be that her cervix was damaged during a previous termination), it does not help to apportion blame or to encourage a woman to feel as if she is the guilty party. This can be a very difficult conversation for you to have with a couple. The woman's partner may do his best to insist that none of this was her fault, but too much insistence can become trying and may sound as if he 'doth protest too much'. Privately he may blame her past (in which he was probably not present) for what has happened. Whatever the situation, as the professional you have to try to do your best to talk about the subject honestly but kindly, using language with care and without suggesting fault, blame or divine judgement.

The Royal College of Obstetricians and Gynaecologists discusses these issues clearly in its guideline on the management of women who suffer miscarriages, quoting a paper by Chalmers from 1992, saying that 'when talking to women, the inadvertent use of inappropriate terms such as "pregnancy failure", or "incompetent cervix" can contribute to negative self-perceptions and worsen any sense of failure, shame, guilt and insecurity'.[3] Therefore, it is essential that medical personnel do not use these expressions. Furthermore, it would be useful to stop thinking about pregnancy loss in these terms and to practise using the same words that women use to describe their loss.

Nuchal scan versus 12-week scan

Most women, and possibly some members of staff, assume that the nuchal scan and the 12-week scan are the same. In fact, the difference between the two is profound and lies at the heart of how a pregnancy is perceived. A nuchal scan is a screening test to enable the risk of the fetus having Down's syndrome to be calculated, with a view to offering the mother a choice about invasive testing and possible termination of an affected pregnancy. In contrast, a 12-week scan measures the baby and checks that it is alive and an appropriate size for its gestational age. Unless this distinction is made clear to women from the outset, at their booking appointment, what they have viewed as an opportunity to see the baby and get a photograph can become a painful dilemma about risk, needles and the potential end of a pregnancy. Perhaps the booking midwife thought that all this had been explained before, or perhaps she preferred not to embark on a conversation about possible tests and termination; either way, it is not fair to assume without first checking that the woman understands the concept of a 'nuchal scan', with all that this implies.

Women who refuse a nuchal scan are likely to have given the matter considerable thought before arriving at their decision. Some women prefer not to have a screening test and are clear about their choice. However, they may find themselves having a difficult time defending their decision, and may be asked at future appointments how they feel about not knowing the risk of their baby having a chromosomal abnormality. It is important that you accept their decision, even if it is not one shared by the majority.

Termination: using language sensitively

If the woman is choosing to have an 'abortion', we should not use the word. If a pregnancy is deliberately ended, for whatever reason, we should use the word 'termination' instead.

A definition of 'abortion' is 'the deliberate termination of a human pregnancy'.[1] It does not help that one of the standard definitions of miscarriage until recent years was 'spontaneous abortion', a phrase used to distinguish a miscarriage from a termination. The word 'abortion' is also used in some quarters to describe something badly done: the *Oxford English Dictionary* defines a second meaning of the word abortion as 'an object or undertaking that is unpleasant or badly made or carried out'.[1] Worse still, until recently, women who suffered repeated miscarriages were told that they had a condition called 'habitual abortion', making it sound as if their losses were somehow due to carelessness, a feckless nature or lack of character.

Before any termination is carried out, two doctors are required to sign the HSA1 form or Certificate A (often called 'the blue form'), which is clearly headed 'ABORTION ACT 1967' in bold and underlined. Similarly, the HSA4 form completed by the doctor who has carried out the termination is clearly headed 'ABORTION NOTIFICATION' in large bold capitals. The first of these forms, by definition, will be in the woman's notes before the procedure begins and the second is often placed there by administrative staff so that the doctor can complete and send it as soon as the procedure is over. It is kind to hide these forms from the woman if this is practicable, since the headings are so visible and unforgiving, especially in cases of therapeutic termination, where women may be insulted by the term.

When miscarriage means termination

Picture a woman who has had an intrauterine fetal death (IUFD) at 15 weeks' gestation, discovered perhaps during a routine scan. Then picture a woman who has preterm spontaneous rupture of her membranes at 15 weeks' gestation and her baby is still alive. After a discussion with senior medical staff, this second woman learns that the outlook for her baby is very grave, since if the pregnancy continues both she and the baby will be susceptible to infection and the fetal lungs will not develop and grow in the context of anhydramnios. Both women may be offered mifepristone and misoprostol to help to 'empty' the uterus. In the case of the first woman, this will be an induced miscarriage. In the case of the second woman, it will be a termination of pregnancy (TOP), since the procedure will start with the fetus still alive *in utero*. Whilst the pharmacological and mechanical processes for each woman are the same, the ethical and legal details are different. It is important that all concerned are aware of the differences, partly so that they can explain honestly to the woman what is about to happen and partly so that they can understand the kinds of feelings that arise in both circumstances. The first woman's baby has died and she may experience the helplessness of her baby dying in circumstances beyond her control. In the second scenario, the woman has to make a decision to end the life of her baby, and whilst what has happened is also beyond her control, uppermost in her mind is that she will be responsible for terminating the life of her baby. What has occurred in the first scenario means the woman was passive in the death of her baby, which is a difficult thing to come to terms with. The woman in the second scenario has to be active in ending her pregnancy. Both are dreadful experiences. The second situation also requires that those staff with conscientious objections to termination of pregnancy absent themselves from the process.

In the first case, the baby is already dead and in the second case the baby will die as a result of medical intervention. As well as having an understanding of their individual experiences of loss, both women will need sympathy, kindness, privacy and pain relief. In the first case, there may be discussions about a post-mortem (PM) examination and blood tests to try to determine why the death occurred. In the second case, two doctors will need to sign the HSA1 form before the procedure begins, and the doctor prescribing the mifepristone will need to complete the HSA4 form afterwards. Swabs may be taken from the placenta and the woman's vagina to try to diagnose whether an infection was the reason for the membrane rupture. The first woman may wonder whether anything she did caused the baby to die. The second woman will know that she agreed to end her baby's life, even though in the circumstances it was the safest and kindest thing to do. Staff members will often share this ambivalence when dealing with cases where a therapeutic termination is performed. In a case like this, though, 'therapeutic termination' is an apposite phrase – the termination is therapeutic for the mother (preventing her from developing sepsis and from having to deal with the loss of her baby at a later gestation), although it is not of course therapeutic for the baby, except in the sense of being a merciful killing. Some members of staff will find this difficult to accept, even if they do not object to termination per se, and will not wish to participate. Others will feel that it is the best thing to do and wish that there were something more that could be done to help the pregnancy continue safely. Others will be pragmatic and practical and feel sure that what is being done is for the best. These differing attitudes and responses are not dissimilar to those that pregnant women and their partners experience.

FIRST TRIMESTER LOSSES

'Early' miscarriage

Having an early miscarriage is a common experience. Despite this, we find that the thought that something might go wrong hardly ever crosses an individual woman's mind. If she does think of it, the thought is not often perceived as being a real possibility, despite the statistics that show that up to one in four women who get pregnant will have a miscarriage.[4] It is important to understand that what we know about something is completely separate from how we experience it. Knowing something for a fact does not in any way imply that you can anticipate how you will deal with it emotionally.

These days, it is easy to do a pregnancy test soon after conception and many women begin to get attached to their pregnancy and the idea of their baby very quickly. Therefore, the end of a pregnancy signalled by the onset of spotting or bleeding can be very difficult for many women. What in the past may have been thought of as a heavy period will now be recognised as a miscarriage. Bleeding is evidence of the loss: it can be both physically and mentally painful and there is no way that a woman who has done an early pregnancy test can be unaware of what is happening.

Women who experience a miscarriage in the first trimester need care and kindness just as much as someone who has a later loss. Each couple needs a response appropriate to their experience of the end of the pregnancy. Patients' reactions to an early loss vary and need to be understood within the context of each person's story. It is important to consider, among other things, how the mother is reacting, whether this is her first pregnancy and how long she had been trying to conceive.

Many hospitals have an early pregnancy assessment unit (EPAU) where women can go if they have pain or bleeding in the first trimester. It means that they can go and get practical information and emotional support when something unexpected is happening. In some hospitals this will be a walk-in service, whereas in others the woman will require a referral from her general practitioner (GP) or another doctor. Most EPAUs will have a sonographer so that viability scans can be performed straight away. The sonographer may be available only for a limited time each day and there may not be an out-of-hours service, in which case the woman would be managed via the accident and emergency department.

Missed miscarriage

A missed miscarriage is often only discovered at the 12-week or nuchal scan, but may also be discovered at a later date. It can be traumatising to be going for a scan, looking forward to receiving confirmation that all is well with the pregnancy, only to be told that the baby has died some time earlier. To have had no indication of this fact often leaves the woman disconcerted and she may have feelings about her body betraying her. It may also be psychologically challenging because she and her partner will have been planning for the rest of her pregnancy, but all the while the pregnancy had ended. Other family members may already know about the pregnancy or the couple may have been planning to announce their news following the scan. If the pregnancy is known about by more people than the individual woman or the couple then there will have to be conversations about the death of the baby. If the news of the baby was going to be given following the scan then the loss may feel more private, but it can be difficult to let people know that you were pregnant and now are not. Even more isolating, as some women choose to do, is to keep the loss of the pregnancy to themselves, and attempt to carry on as if nothing has happened.

Once a diagnosis of a missed miscarriage is given, women are faced with making a decision about what to do: to wait for the baby to 'come away' naturally or to have a procedure to remove the baby. For some women, it is right that they wait for their body to expel the pregnancy, whilst others will want there to be an end as quickly as possible, feeling that as their body has not functioned as they expected they cannot bear to wait. If this is the case, then the ERPC should be made available as soon as possible, ideally later the same day. The procedure is usually done under a general anaesthetic (GA). Sometimes there can be a feeling of unreality for these women, as they have had no physical experience of their loss, unlike a spontaneous miscarriage in which there is pain and bleeding.

More than one miscarriage

If someone is unfortunate enough to have two miscarriages, in our opinion it changes so many of the attitudes that women and their partners have towards pregnancy. Having been brave enough to get pregnant again, for it to go wrong a second time can bring about feelings of desolation and, for some women, a sense of hopelessness. Women and their partners wonder what they have to do to stay pregnant, and given that there is nothing they can do, they are often very frustrated. If the woman does not already have a child, she can be left wondering if she will ever have one. It is terribly important to listen to what women tell you about their thoughts and feelings. It is essential that you do not try to reassure them that everything will be okay, as they are likely to feel dismissed and not believe you.

To have one miscarriage or even two is a common experience, so much so that it is not seen as necessary to investigate the cause of miscarriage until someone has had three. This can seem very cruel for women who have had two losses, but it is perfectly possible to have two consecutive miscarriages and then a successful pregnancy, though not many women will have faith in that being the case. The term used after three miscarriages is 'recurrent miscarriage'.

Once a couple is in this category, tests will be carried out to try to establish any cause. Whilst patients are generally keen to be tested, they are anxious about the possible results of the tests. On one hand they want something to be wrong, so that it can be fixed and they can have a successful pregnancy, but on the other hand there is a reluctance to acknowledge that if there is a problem it might be someone's (usually the woman's) fault. The tests may also reveal that there is no obvious reason for the miscarriages, which may make patients feel despondent about not being able to fix anything.

When couples consider another pregnancy, there may be a difference in the way the partners react: one may be desperate to try again as soon as possible and the other may feel that a break and a rest may be a good idea. Some women or their partners might even feel that it would be too stressful to risk going through another pregnancy and not want to embark on one at all.

Ectopic pregnancy

An 'ectopic pregnancy' is a complication of pregnancy in which the embryo implants outside the womb. Ectopic pregnancies are not usually viable and they can be dangerous because internal bleeding can occur and become a life-threatening complication. Most arise in the fallopian tube, but implantation can also occur in the cervix, ovaries and abdomen. Being able to detect an early ectopic pregnancy has become easier due to enhanced diagnostic capability and many are now managed medically. The introduction of methotrexate treatment for ectopic pregnancy has reduced the need for surgery, but surgical intervention is still required in cases where the fallopian tube has ruptured or is in danger of doing so. This will mean that the woman will need either a laparoscopy or a laparotomy.

An ectopic pregnancy is a potential medical emergency that can be fatal if not treated properly. This can be difficult for women to appreciate. They may often be in the early stages of pregnancy and find it hard to be told that their pregnancy needs to end and that they are at risk of dying if it does not. Psychologically, it can be helpful if they at least have some pain as a warning sign, otherwise they are in the position of having to trust what they are being told.

When surgery is required, it can seem a dramatic and drastic step. It is important to talk to the woman and her partner both before and after the procedure, as she is likely to be in psychological, and possibly physical, shock. Women may find it very hard to believe that their pregnancy is over and may ask about transplanting the ectopic pregnancy into the womb so that it can continue. This is not possible and women need to be told this, preferably before their operation, so that there is no misunderstanding.

We have known women who have come to hospital, with or sometimes without pain, and within a few hours are in theatre, with their pregnancy ended and a fallopian tube removed. The impact of this situation takes some time to absorb; not only have they lost a baby but they have had surgery, too. Because of the shock and the need for urgent intervention, it is useful for women who have had surgical removal of an ectopic pregnancy to have a follow-up appointment with a consultant within 6 weeks of the procedure. As well as the loss of the baby, there may be a significant impact on their fertility. Women usually imagine that losing a tube will halve their chances of becoming pregnant in the future. Statistics about this are difficult to analyse, but it may be that the chances are not so severely reduced, since it is possible to conceive via one tube with an egg from the opposite ovary. Success in a future pregnancy will depend largely on the state of the remaining tube, which should be noted by the surgeon during the operation and then discussed with the woman.

Diagnosis of fetal abnormality

Most (but not all) women will have a nuchal translucency scan, which may be combined with serum screening, at about 12 weeks' gestation, to screen for Down's syndrome. If a result is deemed 'screen positive', the woman will be offered further investigations, either chorionic villus sampling (CVS) or amniocentesis to confirm the fetal chromosome pattern. If this test proves that the fetus has an abnormal karyotype, the woman will be given the option of a TOP. It is important to see that there are choices available at each step of this process. Just because a woman opts for a nuchal scan does not necessarily mean that she will choose to terminate a pregnancy with an abnormal karyotype. She may prefer to see the tests as a way of preparing herself for what is to come when her child is born. Other women will be sure that they do not want a child with a chromosomal abnormality: they may want to bypass the screening stage and go straight to an invasive diagnostic test, sure that they will go for termination if the result confirms their fears.

The anomalies commonly diagnosed by amniocentesis or CVS are the most frequently occurring of the trisomies: trisomy 21 (Down's syndrome), trisomy 18 (Edwards' syndrome) and trisomy 13 (Patau's syndrome), and sickle cell disease in pregnancies in which both parents have sickle cell trait.

Therapeutic TOP will usually involve the use of a version of prostaglandin to induce a miscarriage, often preceded by a dose of the anti-progesterone mifepristone. Once the prostaglandin starts to be administered, the process of labour and delivery may take many hours or even days, especially in a first pregnancy. Careful consideration must be given to pain relief: some women will want to be clear and alert throughout the process and may want an epidural, whereas others may want to be somewhat sedated and will prefer a patient-controlled analgesia (PCA) system that will allow them to dispense their own morphine. Use of either an epidural or PCA necessitates one-to-one care from a midwife who has been specifically trained in their use. Maternity managers will usually liaise with their anaesthetic colleagues to provide this training.

If the pregnancy to be terminated has reached 22 weeks, feticide is recommended to prevent the possibility of the baby being born alive,[5] which would be extremely distressing for both the parents and the attending staff. Feticide will be performed by a fetal medicine specialist, usually prior to the woman's admission to hospital, and involves a scan to visualise the fetal heart and then the injection of potassium chloride into one of the cardiac chambers.

The organisation Antenatal Results and Choices (ARC)[6] is a national charity that provides non-directive support and information to parents throughout and after the antenatal screening and diagnostic process. ARC is extremely useful for both parents and staff, and any couple facing difficult decisions regarding an abnormal fetus will find ARC's literature and support helpful.

Parents who choose a therapeutic TOP for fetal abnormality vary when it comes to the decision about whether to ask for a PM examination on the baby. Some will feel that they know the baby's diagnosis from the scans and tests and that a PM is not necessary. Others will find a PM useful in that it will (hopefully) confirm the diagnosis and help to vindicate their decision to end the pregnancy. It is important to help parents reach their conclusion about this in their own time and in their own way, rather than suggest what you think is the right decision.

As we have already said, problems with the way a baby is developing are usually diagnosed either at the nuchal scan or the 20-week anomaly scan. Despite women having been given literature regarding the screening purpose of scans, most of them will manage to disassociate themselves from the information and believe that their baby is bound to be normal. For those who discover that there is something wrong with the way their baby is developing, either a chromosomal or developmental problem, it can be devastating. They are facing a problem they have not expected and are faced with having to decide what to do next. Some will be certain, either from the moment of diagnosis or after consideration, that they will carry on with the pregnancy – either to see if nature takes its course and the pregnancy ends naturally or because they want their baby to be born (even knowing that she might die shortly after birth) and are prepared to bring up a child who has some form of disability. Women who reach a decision to terminate their pregnancy need support and recognition of the dilemma they are dealing with. If women decide to continue with a pregnancy they need additional support from experienced staff.

Finding themselves in this position is complicated and long after reaching a decision, women may continue to wonder if they have made the correct one. Recently, we met a woman who with each pregnancy has a statistical chance of her baby having a heart problem, which means that he will die within months of birth. At a follow-up meeting to discuss her most recent decision to terminate her pregnancy she declared that she would never be tested for this problem in any future pregnancy. Her first baby had been born before the condition was known and he had died at 5 months. She said that she would rather go through the pain of her baby dying after birth than have another termination. Fortunately, not many women are faced with this particular patient's problem, but it highlights some of the dilemmas involved, and just how impossible it is to get it right. In these situations, it may help you to not think about a patient getting it right or wrong but merely about her making the best decision she can in an impossible situation. In our experience, when women or couples are further away from the immediacy of the decision, they may regret what they opted for and it can be useful to remind them gently of their emotional, mental and physical reality at the time of their dilemma. In the remembering, they can be reassured that they probably could not have done anything differently.

It is vital that staff have some idea of what it feels like to have to decide to end the life of a baby or to carry on with a pregnancy after a diagnosis of abnormality. It is essential that we as professionals adopt a non-judgemental position and have an unconditional positive regard for couples in this situation. Unconditional positive regard means accepting people for who they are without disapproving of feelings, actions or characteristics, regardless of whether you agree with them. It also means having the ability to listen without interrupting or making judgements, as well as not giving your own opinion or advice. All those faced with such decisions will consider what to do carefully. Some will reach their decision in a short space of time, others agonise over what to do and need time to decide. Either way, people may have to end a wanted pregnancy or alter the dreams they had regarding their perfect baby. If the pregnancy was initially not desired, it can be an even harder decision as the individual or couple have their early ambivalence to contend with as well as deciding whether to continue the pregnancy. People rarely expect to find themselves in this difficult position. They will have been given, and have possibly taken notice of, the statistical odds of there being a problem with their baby, but what they quickly learn is that statistics are only useful as long as you are not the one out of the tens, hundreds or thousands quoted. If you are singled out in this way, then you lose forever the cushion of safety that statistics give the majority, who are fortunate enough never to have to address being the 'one'.

Molar pregnancy

For some women, a first trimester scan will show a hydatidiform mole rather than an ongoing pregnancy with a live fetus. Usually, molar pregnancies present before 12 weeks with severe hyperemesis gravidarum. A mole is a disease of the trophoblast, or developing placental tissue, that results from the egg being fertilised by too many sperm. There is no choice other than to terminate the pregnancy, and there is the added issue of the possibility of developing gestational trophoblastic disease. This involves prolonged follow-up of the woman's beta human chorionic gonadotrophin levels and possible cytotoxic treatment before she can safely try to conceive again. Not only must these women contend with discovering that they were never really pregnant in the conventional sense of the word, but that they have also developed a potentially serious condition that requires careful management. Finding themselves in this situation can make them feel that their body has let them down and fooled them. The extended follow-up after a molar pregnancy can actually help women to regain a sense of trust about their body, as most of them do not develop the disease.

SECOND TRIMESTER LOSS

Miscarriage in the second trimester can be both physically and mentally taxing. Whilst something going wrong after the first trimester is rarer, it is not unusual from the obstetric point of view. Most people tend to think of miscarriage as happening within the first 12 weeks of pregnancy. They feel safe having got past that time. It is important to recognise that second trimester losses occur during what could be called the 'quiet' time of pregnancy: morning sickness has stopped, usually there are no scans to check on the baby's progress and it is too early for the woman to experience the baby's movements very much.

Second trimester loss can occur as a miscarriage with bleeding and painful uterine contractions or result from a 'weak' cervix, with the loss being typically sudden and painless. Other losses will result from premature rupture of the membranes or late missed miscarriages.

Between the gestation ages of 12 and 16 weeks, if the miscarriage has not come away naturally, the woman will need to decide how to proceed. She may be given the choice of a surgical procedure such as an ERPC or having an induced miscarriage – giving birth. Giving birth may well be a frightening idea, so you need to talk her and her partner about what this means. Usually she will go to a ward where staff who are experienced in working with women and pregnancy loss need to be available. This may be a gynaecology ward or a separate part of a women's surgical ward. More rarely, this will be on a labour ward but away from the sound of labouring women.

Mid-trimester losses include babies of up to 24 weeks' gestation. Prior to 20 weeks, most women are comfortable with their loss being described as a 'late miscarriage'. However, once women reach 20 weeks and beyond, especially if they have to give birth to their baby, they find the term 'miscarriage' lessens the meaning of their loss. They want words that describe the seriousness of their loss. This is not only important for them but also for all those with whom they have contact. They want their friends and work colleagues to know the significance of what they have been through and that they have not 'just had a miscarriage'. It can feel especially cruel that if your baby died at 23 weeks and 6 days you are classified as having had a 'miscarriage', whereas if your baby had lived for another day you would be described as having had a 'stillbirth'. You are not entitled to maternity leave in the former situation, whereas in the latter you are. It is very hard to live with this demarcation and women do not like it.

Therapeutic termination of pregnancy

Termination for severe fetal abnormality is allowed under clause E of the Abortion Act 1967 (UK), without any limit on the gestational age at which the procedure is carried out. This means that a relatively small number of terminations are carried out after 24 weeks' gestation, almost always with a preceding feticide so that the baby is not born alive. This actually means that the baby's heart has to be stopped and this can be a terrible decision for parents to have to make. Recently, a couple at the follow-up perinatal loss clinic said that they wished that they had not been asked for their consent, as they found this the worst part of the experience. Whilst there is absolutely no way that they could have been exempted from the decision, it is easy to sympathise with their desire not to be responsible for stopping the life of their baby. This is an acutely painful dilemma and patients may need you to let them talk about their feelings and their reasons for opting for a termination.

Whilst there are often logical reasons for the 'delay' in carrying out these terminations, such as diagnosing a very poor prognosis after monitoring a pregnancy with a major abnormality for several weeks, there is inevitably a discomfort felt by staff attending these cases, even if they understand intellectually and agree with what is happening. Debates in the medical press regarding the management of fetal pain and whether allowing very late termination for fetal abnormality is discriminatory only add to any existing ambivalence that staff may feel.[7]

In some ways, staff have to learn to disconnect their attitudes towards looking after someone who at 23 weeks is losing a baby that there may be a chance of saving, from those towards feticide and termination at a similar gestation. It is quite possible that within the same maternity unit at the same time there will be women going through both experiences. It is only natural to feel the irony here. On one hand we strive to save a tiny preterm baby in the hope that he will beat the odds and survive unharmed, whilst on the other hand we calculate that another baby would be better dead than alive and so set about ending his life. It is understandable that staff who spend much of their working lives trying to save very preterm babies (i.e. doctors and nurses from the neonatal unit) will feel uncomfortable about the thought of late termination, and may express their discomfort to their obstetric colleagues. Just because you feel discomfort does not mean that you are wrong or right. Your feelings are genuine and you should not deny them. For you they are valid and it is important to acknowledge them, as long as they do not affect the care you give to patients. Learning to deal with both situations calmly and professionally falls to the staff on the maternity unit who must be able to flip from one case to the other in a matter of minutes. You need to be able to use the same empathy, knowledge and mental ability in both situations. The ability of each staff member to compartmentalise his or her mind so that work and life outside of work are separated is called into play when dealing with cases like this.

Some women will want to wait for their baby to die, perhaps despite medical concern about their own health, and will feel relieved when she dies naturally and they did not have to decide to end the pregnancy themselves. Sometimes this process can take weeks, for example, if a baby has severe intrauterine growth restriction. Women and their partners need to be given ongoing support whilst they wait for this to happen. They need regular scans to monitor what is happening to the baby and may need emotional help whilst coming to terms with waiting for their baby's death.

EDGES OF VIABILITY

A baby is 'live born' if he shows 'signs of life' once delivered. All definitions of the term use the plural, 'signs' of life rather than a 'sign' of life. Any baby born alive who dies within a week will be classified as a live birth and a neonatal death. A baby born with signs of life before 24 completed weeks' gestation is live born, and if he dies this will be a neonatal death rather than a stillbirth or a miscarriage, regardless of the baby's gestational age at birth. The importance of trying to have a doctor present at the birth of infants at the edges of viability, in case there are signs of life, is discussed more fully in Chapter 10 in relation to completing the relevant certificates.

One of the main reasons to be accurate about gestational age and expected date of delivery (EDD) is so that if a woman threatens to deliver very prematurely one can be clear about how the baby may be managed. The EDD can be calculated from the first day of the last menstrual period using Naegele's rule (add nine calendar months plus a week) as long as the woman has a regular 28-day cycle and is certain of the date of her last period. Usually, the EDD will be calculated using measurements from an early dating scan and confirmed at the 20-week anomaly scan. Once confirmed, there should be no argument, either from patients or staff, about the EDD. It is certainly not appropriate to start arguing about the EDD when a woman is about to deliver a very preterm baby. We have had experience of couples debating the EDD with members of staff when the woman is about to deliver very prematurely, in an attempt to make their baby 'older' than she really is. This is understandable, as the parents wish to try to give their baby every possible chance of survival, but their efforts may be misjudged at best and must be gently prevented if at all possible.

For example, if a woman is about to deliver a baby at 24 weeks and 2 days, it would be reasonable to predict that the baby may be born alive and may respond to resuscitation, since his lungs are formed and theoretically capable of being inflated. If a woman is about to deliver at 22 weeks and 2 days, the lungs are not yet properly formed and resuscitation efforts will be fruitless. Two weeks is a long time in the life of an unborn baby at this gestation. Even if the latter baby is born showing signs of life (for example, she has a heartbeat and she makes gasping movements), she will not be able to survive, since it will not be possible for her lungs to be ventilated. Instead, she should be made comfortable to die peacefully in her mother's arms if this is what she and her partner want. Staff need to be able to talk to couples about what to expect and to prepare them before the birth of their baby. Couples have told us about how precious it was for them to spend time with their baby even though they knew he would die.

We have known of very preterm babies being resuscitated against the better judgement of the neonatal and obstetric staff because of parental insistence about the gestational age, only for their baby to die soon afterwards in very upsetting circumstances. This is made obvious, for example, by the monitoring equipment usually employed to help babies in the neonatal unit, which is too harsh for the incredibly thin skin of a baby delivered at 22 weeks, causing burns and sores.

In most units in the UK, the neonatal team will not attend the delivery of a baby under 23 weeks' gestation. This makes it clear to both parents and maternity staff that it is not appropriate to try to resuscitate a baby that is too premature to be able to survive. Attendance at deliveries for babies of 23 weeks and over does not necessarily mean that resuscitation will be attempted; this will depend on the condition of the baby at birth and whether she shows any signs of life. This varies between countries: the EURONIC Project,[8] which looked at practice in various European countries, found that in The Netherlands resuscitation will not be attempted until the baby has reached 25 or 26 weeks' gestation. As well as variation between countries in terms of resuscitation according to gestational age, there were also differences in other aspects of end-of-life decision-making.[9]

THIRD TRIMESTER LOSS
Stillbirth

The medical definition of a 'stillborn' baby is one that is delivered without signs of life after 24 completed weeks' gestation. A stillbirth may arise because of an intrauterine death before labour or because of the baby's death during labour. Some practitioners make a distinction between an intrauterine death (meaning death before labour) and a stillbirth (by which they mean that the death occurred during labour), but this can lead to unnecessary confusion.

Strictly speaking, one should say 'intrapartum stillbirth' if the death occurred during labour.

The *Oxford English Dictionary* definition of 'stillbirth' is 'the birth of an infant that has died in the womb (strictly, after having survived through at least the first 28 weeks of pregnancy, earlier instances being regarded as abortion or miscarriage)'.[1] The different gestational age is interesting and reflects the fact that, until fairly recently, a baby was considered unviable if born prior to 28 weeks. It was also the case that until 1990 the legal time limit for termination of pregnancy in the UK (other than under clause E) was 28 weeks. The legal time limit was lowered to 24 weeks with the 1990 amendment, since by then 24 weeks was considered the age of fetal viability.

Intrauterine death

The range of third trimester loss is from 26 weeks' gestation to full term. Having reached 26 weeks or further along in their pregnancies, most women begin to feel confident about their expectations of having a baby. They will have had a number of weeks during which they will have felt their baby move. An IUFD is usually first noticed by a reduction or cessation of movement. Alternatively, it will be recognised at a routine midwifery appointment, when the midwife cannot locate the baby's heartbeat. As we said earlier, the death will be classified as a stillbirth or an IUFD. This fact, at least, gives some indication of the significance and seriousness of the death. Other people will understand from the terminology that a baby has died, rather than the woman having had a miscarriage, which often does not conjure the reality of a baby in some people's minds. A baby dying after the age of viability is truly devastating; there is the thought of 'if only she had been born a day earlier she would be here with me now'. Certainly that is sometimes the case, but in other situations it emerges over time that no matter when the baby had been born, he would not have survived. Parents feel the helplessness of not being able to change what has happened, as well as facing the stark reality of their baby being dead. To have got so close to having a baby, only for their baby to die, is cruel. It may be helpful to think of the implications of the death as being like a stone thrown into a pool: there are ripples, some nearer the centre, which would represent the parents, and then as they widen out they represent the effect on all the other people involved in the patient's life. This will include existing children and grandparents.

Intrapartum stillbirth

The number of babies that actually die during labour is low. This information will not help those who are unfortunate enough to have started labour with a live baby only to finish labour with a baby that has died. Intrapartum still-birth may occur for various reasons including a placental abruption, a true knot in the umbilical cord or hypoxia. It is a shattering experience for all those involved, including the staff. For the parents, it is likely to be an overwhelm-ing and shocking incident with lifelong consequences.

Early neonatal death

A 'neonatal death' is defined as one occurring within the first 28 days of life. An 'early neonatal death' is one that occurs in the first 7 days of life. This means that those deaths that occur very soon after the birth will be classi-fied as early neonatal deaths. This will include very preterm babies born alive before 24 weeks but who die soon after birth. Giving birth to a premature baby or a baby who is ill becomes a whole different experience. Instead of leaving hospital with your baby, mothers and fathers have to become familiar with a neonatal ward and all that this involves. Neonatal staff have to be aware of the language they use and how their descriptions of the baby's condition are being understood by the parents. Telling a parent that their (sick) baby is 'doing well' could mean that the parent will hear this as if you are talking about a fit baby and they will be optimistic about their baby's survival. Really, the sub-context is 'given how poorly your baby is, he is doing well by managing to stay alive'. If parents are not given realistic information about their baby's condition, they can end up being surprised and devastated when he dies. When it becomes clear that it is better and kinder for the baby to withdraw life support, parents need to be prepared in advance for this event. Many will want to be present; it may be that it is only after the withdrawal that they can hold him for the first time. Suitable private places need to be available for parents to spend as much time as they want with their baby during this process.

TWINS

Twin pregnancies (and higher multiples) are defined by their chorionicity, which will usually be determined at an early scan. The risk of pregnancy loss varies with different types of twins. Dichorionic diamniotic (DCDA) twins have separate placentae and separate sacs. Most are dizygotic (non-identical), and they have the lowest complication rate of all twin pregnancies. Monochorionic diamniotic (MCDA) twins are almost always monozygotic (identical). They share a placenta but have separate amniotic sacs. Monochorionic monoamniotic (MCMA) twins are always monozygotic and share a placenta and an amniotic sac. For this reason their cords can become very entangled, resulting in a higher mortality rate than other types of twins.

A twin pregnancy is known to be a complicated pregnancy and the death of one or both twins is a real possibility. As well as being complicated, it is also special to be pregnant with twins and for both twins to die is a double blow. There is an additional aspect of loss for those parents whose identical twins die, as they know that the possibility of being pregnant again with another set of twins is highly unlikely. The grief following the loss of twins conceived with in vitro fertilisation (IVF) is heightened because the possibility of another pregnancy resulting in a baby is so much more daunting or may seem impossible.

If the twin pregnancy was the first pregnancy, it means that by the time the couple actually has a live baby they will have been parents to three children. This is challenging to manage. The death of twins needs to be given the same kind of respect as the death of a singleton baby and you need to be aware of the significance of the double loss to parents. When talking to them about their loss, you need to be careful to refer to both babies, either by name or by saying 'the girls', for example.

There are various types of twin losses; these are discussed below.

Vanishing twin syndrome

The phenomenon of the vanishing twin has been recognised since the increase in the use of ultrasound scans early in pregnancy. A scan at 6 weeks may show two gestation sacs but a scan later in the pregnancy will show only one fetus, the other having been resorbed. The survivors of vanishing twin pregnancies may be at higher risk of being small for gestational age than other singletons,[10] but most survivors of vanishing twin syndrome are unknown because many twins vanish without their mothers or midwives being aware that this has happened.

They die one after the other

This may happen if a woman miscarries one twin and the pregnancy continues, only for the second twin to be miscarried later. It occurs, for example, when there is preterm membrane rupture of the first sac, causing the loss of the first twin, and subsequent chorioamnionitis affecting the second sac.

Both die at the same time

There is a higher incidence of loss in twin pregnancies than in singleton pregnancies. The risk is highest with MCMA twins[11] and is higher in MCDA twins than in DCDA twins.[12]

Twin-to-twin transfusion syndrome (TTTS)

Monochorionic twins may have an anastomosis between the blood vessels in a shared part of their placenta, so that blood can pass from one twin to the other. The donor twin's growth becomes restricted and the recipient twin becomes bigger. TTTS will be diagnosed when serial ultrasound scans show a discrepancy between the twins' sizes. Both twins are at risk from unrecognised TTTS, one from intrauterine growth restriction and the other from cardiac failure.

One twin dies and the other survives and the pregnancy continues

This can happen with DCDA twins, since they each have a separate placenta and are independent of each other. Depending on when the death occurred, the dead fetus may become shrivelled and flat by the time of the delivery (a so-called fetus papyraceus) or may be more recognisably a baby but macerated.

One version of this type of loss occurs if one twin is diagnosed with a severe abnormality and the mother elects to have selective feticide of the affected twin and allow the pregnancy to continue with the healthy twin as a singleton. If this is done with dichorionic twins, usually by injecting intra-cardiac potassium chloride, the risk of loss of the remaining twin is about 10% with first trimester feticide and half that with later procedures. Selective feticide in monochorionic twin pregnancies is carried out with bipolar umbilical cord diathermy and is safer if carried out at later gestations. An Australian review of 118 cases reported an overall survival rate for the remaining twin of 71%.[13]

It is a genuinely taxing experience to be celebrating the live birth of one of your babies and mourning the death of the other. There is in fact very little chance of celebrating, but rather there is relief that one baby has survived and immense sadness at the other's death. Not only do parents become conscious of their loss, but they will also be acutely aware of the loss for the remaining baby. They no longer have their womb companion and they will be forever bereft and deprived of their company. Parents are thrown into all that goes with being a mother (and father) with one of their babies but have to deal with all the grief associated with not having the other. There is then the worry that grieving is affecting the live baby. Additionally, women report how scared they are for some considerable time. They are frightened that something will happen to the surviving baby and that he, too, might die. This is especially so if the baby has had to be in the neonatal unit for any length of time. This is entirely normal and you can help as a caregiver by being empathic and supportive. It is really important, too, that staff involved in looking after parents who are in this situation help them create as many memories and mementoes of both babies as possible. Can the parents hold both twins together? Is it possible to take a picture of the twins together as well as with the parents holding them? It is also hugely important that once the babies are separated that staff do not talk about surviving twins as if they are a singleton babies, as this will be hurtful and seem dismissive of the parents' experience.

Once parents have left the hospital and re-entered the outside world, they will look like a couple with a baby, which of course they are, but it will not occur to many people that they are also dealing with being robbed of having both of their children. Explaining this to people can become a chore and an additional burden, but parents will never want to deny the existence of all of their babies. If you are seeing parents once they are at home, it is imperative that you ask them how they are managing with the complexities of their parenting and their grieving. The situation they are in is for life and you can help them by acknowledging their total experience. Just as the loss of a single baby gives parents a heightened awareness of pregnant women and small babies, twins will now seem to be everywhere and this can a be difficult and painful reminder of what they have lost.

One of the ongoing issues for the bereaved parents of one twin is how to include their deceased child whilst the survivor grows up and away from the time that they had the experience of being a twin. Birthdays can be fraught if some thought is not given to how to make it okay for the survivor as well as acknowledging the love for the deceased twin. We know of a couple who, in order to separate the birthday of their surviving twin from that of the one who died *in utero*, commemorate her existence on the day that they found out that she had died. This way both twins can have a special day. It also means that the baby boy who survived can honour his sister throughout his life and he is aware that he is a twin. This is not always the case for those people whose twin died before they could be born. It is increasingly understood that even if people are aware that they have been a twin, there are common feelings that something is missing from their lives and parents will need to acknowledge this, just as it is the case for them. They may also wonder why they survived and their sibling did not. Parents and twin survivors have to contend with these and other psychological implications, and be given help if they need it.

SUMMARY

This chapter demonstrates the variety of pregnancy losses and illustrates the large number of problems women and their families may encounter. We want to stress that the emotional impact of the experience is not necessarily dependent on the gestation at which the loss occurs and staff must be prepared to be supportive and helpful in all cases.

REFERENCES

1. *Oxford English Dictionary*. Available at: www.oxforddictionaries.com/words/the-oxford-english-dictionary (accessed 26 August 2012).
2. *Collins Thesaurus*. Available at: www.collinsdictionary.com/english-thesaurus (accessed 26 August 2012).
3. Chalmers B. Terminology used in early pregnancy loss. *Br J Obstet Gynaecol.* 1992; **99**(5): 357–8.
4. Regan L. *Miscarriage: what every woman needs to know.* London: Bloomsbury Publishing; 1997.
5. Royal College of Obstetricians and Gynaecologists (RCOG). *The Care of Women Requesting Induced Abortion.* Evidence-based Clinical Guideline Number 7. London: RCOG Press; 2011. Available at: www.rcog.org.uk/files/rcog-corp/Abortion%20guideline_web_1.pdf (accessed 17 August 2012).
6. www.arc-uk.org
7. Statham H, Solomou W, Green J. Late termination of pregnancy: law, policy and decision making in four English fetal medicine units. *BJOG.* 2006; **113**(12): 1402–11.
8. Cuttini M, Nadai M, Kaminski M *et al.* End-of-life decisions in neonatal intensive care: physicians' self-reported practices in seven European countries. EURONIC Study Group. *Lancet.* 2000; **355**(9221): 2112–18.
9. Baer GR, Nelson RM. A review of ethical issues involved in premature birth. In: Behrman RE, Butler AS, editors. *Preterm Birth: causes, consequences, and prevention.* Washington DC: National Academies Press; 2007: pp. 669–70.
10. Shebl O, Ebner T, Sommergruber M *et al.* Birth weight is lower for survivors of the vanishing twin syndrome: a case-control study. *Fertil Steril.* 2008; **90**(2): 310–14.
11. Rossi AC, D'Addario V. Umbilical cord occlusion for selective feticide in complicated monochorionic twins: a systematic review of literature. *Am J Obstet Gynecol.* 2009; **2**(200): 123–9.
12. Dias, T, Contro E, Thilaganathan B *et al.* Pregnancy outcome of monochorionic twins: does amnionicity matter? *Twin Res Hum Genet.* 2011; **14**(6): 586–92.
13. Lee YM, Wylie BJ, Simpson LL *et al.* Twin chorionicity and the risk of stillbirth. *Obstet Gynecol.* 2008; **111**(2 Pt 1): 301–8.

CHAPTER 3

Bad and sad news

INTRODUCTION

This chapter is about looking at the roles and responsibilities staff have when there is the need to tell a mother and her partner that their baby has died.

Giving difficult information to patients is usually known as 'breaking' bad news. This can be a challenging way to think about your responsibility in the task of telling people something is wrong. Lots of the research into breaking bad news talks about the stress that medical staff feel in having this duty and we think that using the terminology 'breaking bad news' adds to the stress. To 'break' something is to fracture it – something that previously was whole is now damaged. Thus, having the task of delivering bad news described as 'breaking', can make you feel accountable for what is broken, whereas in most circumstances you will not be responsible for the unfortunate events that occur in people's lives, including their baby dying. What you are responsible for is telling someone the sad news that their baby is no longer alive. In our experience, staff often feel that it is a huge responsibility to tell someone that their baby is dead – and so it is. The responsibility makes some people think that they will be blamed for the news; that they, as the messenger, will be shot.

To us, it seems much better and less onerous to think of 'imparting' or 'telling' people sad or bad news. This way, the focus can change from being on the person telling the news to the person receiving it. Whilst it will never be an easy thing to do, it may be that giving bad news can become less stressful for medical personnel.

When giving people difficult information, the person conveying the news actually needs their ego to get out of the way. Telling someone that their baby has died is not about the person imparting the news; it is about the event of the death and how the information about what has occurred is received by the mother and father. Being one of the people who has to tell parents of a loss or problem in a pregnancy requires skill, tact and kindness.

Much of the literature regarding breaking bad news advises 'setting the scene'. Because the discovery of the death or a life-threatening problem will be in the moment and probably highly unexpected (certainly by the mother), it is important that front-line staff are constantly prepared for 'setting the scene'. This is unlike a lot of medical situations in which there has been some pre-amble – for example, a case in which a patient has some investigations into their health and is afterwards given the diagnosis of cancer. In this scenario, there is time to set the scene, but the discovery of a baby's death is usually sudden and there is not time to set the scene in advance.

GIVING BAD NEWS

Staff need to have training and support for this vital role. In a training pack for professionals dealing with pregnancy loss, Kohner and Leftwich[1] have made suggestions regarding the principles involved in giving bad news:

1. Be honest and open
2. Keep the message short and clear
3. Use correct words (like 'dead' or 'death', not euphemisms)
4. Do not overload with information
5. Find the most appropriate place available
6. Give time
7. Be prepared for a range of reactions from silence to extreme distress and anger
8. Be genuine
9. Express sorrow and regret
10. If a second opinion is being sought (for example about a scan) acknowl-edge that the delay might be distressing
11. Get support for yourself from a colleague.

We look at their suggestions in greater detail below, using an order that reflects the circumstances in which bad news would usually be given, rather than the order in the list above.

Being honest and open (1) sounds fairly simple but is actually quite a challenging and skilful task. What is required is that you are composed and have as much information about the situation as possible so that you are prepared for reactions and questions from patients. If you do not know the answer to any questions, tell them that you do not know and that you will either find out or you will get someone who knows the answer to talk to them.

Moreover, it is very important that you make sure you do what you have promised and that you give them a realistic time frame for how long it will take to address their query. What you must not do is guess or tell people something incorrect. Not only will it distress parents once they know that the information was untrue, but it will also make it much more difficult for your colleagues who come after you to correct the mistakes. In addition, it is likely to cause confusion as to who can be trusted.

We know of situations in which women have been told that their baby died because their cervix was weak or because the cord was round the baby's neck. These turned out not to be the causes of death and it was then difficult and distressing for the woman and her family to have to amend their thinking. It may be that there is no known reason for their baby's death, but by giving incorrect information, you raise hopes of an explanation that will later be dashed.

If you are asked a question for which you do not have an answer, at least at the time of being asked, acknowledge that you understand how much they want an answer to their question and that it is frustrating for them to have to wait. For example, you can actually say 'I really wish I could tell you why your baby has died, but at this time it is not clear and I would not want to give you wrong or unhelpful information.' Most patients will understand this.

Getting a second opinion (10) to confirm the baby's death is good practice and it is important to apply some of the other suggestions in the list to explain what you are doing and how long it will take to get someone else. If there is a delay in finding a colleague, acknowledge this and concede that this is an added stress for the mother and her companions.

Keep the message short and clear (2) and use correct words (3). We understand these suggestions to mean that the essential information is that the baby has died and that you need to convey this in the kindest and most unambiguous way: do not say 'I cannot find your baby's heartbeat' if what you mean is 'your baby is dead'. You may inadvertently be setting up an expectation that someone else may be able to find the heartbeat. Instead, you can say 'I'm very sorry to have to tell you some sad news, your baby has died.' Expressing sorrow and regret (9) is appropriate at the time of telling people the bad news. Another way to tell patients would be to say, 'The news is sad, your baby has died, I'm so sorry.'

You then need to be prepared for the patient's reaction to this news. This is where giving time (6) and finding the right place (5) would come in. It is all part of setting the scene, not for actually giving the news, but for managing the impact of the news. If you have told the woman sad news in an ultrasound or consulting room, it may be appropriate to move her to a more suitable room that will ensure her privacy and where she can have as much time as she wants. Additionally, you need to give yourself time for the tasks involved as well as giving time to the patient. You may have to go and let your colleagues know that you will not be available for a while. If the woman came to see you or came to the hospital on her own then it is important to ask her if there is any-one she wants to contact or if she wants you to contact someone on her behalf.

If you are not the most suitable person to carry on looking after her then, once you have got her established in a private room, explain to her that you are going to get a colleague who will look after her and give some indication as to how long that might take. If it takes longer than you have indicated, go back and tell her she is not forgotten.

Reactions to sad or bad news (7) are often similar to initial grief reac-tions: some people will be stunned into silence and some will be angry, hurt or visibly emotional, so you need to be prepared for them and to allow any or a mixture of these responses. Remember, this is the immediate and initial reaction to what is going to be a much longer process. Being accepting of any of these reactions will help patients enormously. We know that for you as a health professional this may be difficult, as you may find yourself wanting to do something to help to make things better.

Doctors and midwives are trained to do something (e.g. to find solutions or ease pain). Being there for people is doing something, but not all medical staff realise this. The guidelines published by Sands[2] mention that

> there is a tendency to react to tears as one does a haemorrhage. However crying is a release, and parents value the support of staff who can cope with their tears without embarrassment. Many people react to bad news and shock with anger and look for someone to blame: this should not be taken personally.

If you can remain calm and support people in their initial reactions of shock, pain and sorrow, you will be doing a huge amount.

Once the news has begun to become a reality, or as part of enabling it to sink in, you can ask people if they want some time to be alone or if they want to go and have a tea or coffee and come back later. Feedback from women who were given the bad news that they had gynaecological cancer was that they wished that the clinic had been run in such a way as to allow them to be told the diagnosis and then for them to go away and come back within the opening time of the clinic. This way, they would have had time to work out what they needed to know and time to formulate their questions.

It is important to offer these suggestions in a manner that makes it clear to patients that they are not being abandoned or that the death of their baby is unbearable for staff.

Most people, whether they are patients or not, can tell if the individuals they meet are genuine (8). Being genuine includes you showing your care as the human being you are rather than hiding behind your professional role, whilst not over-identifying with your patient. In one case, the parents told us that the midwife who was looking after them so over-identified with their loss that she told them 'that if they had had a bad day, she had an even worse one'.

In counselling terms, being genuine goes along with having unconditional positive regard for another person. Having unconditional positive regard for an individual means that you are accepting of that person without any preconceptions about them and that you care about them even if they have traits or ways of managing life that you do not recognise or agree with.

Patients are completely dependent on whom they meet and we currently have a health service in which kindness is not always a prerequisite. Kindness does not often appear in the personnel specification as an essential requirement, so sometimes patients feel cared for and sometimes they feel the opposite. As we have said before, if they are not cared for, it will add insult to the injury of their loss.

> Kindness is a concept that is sometimes experienced within the institutions but is not a held, and supported and empowered value within them. So, in a hospital, it is there if there are kind nurses or doctors on duty and not there if there are unkind or neutral people.[3]

Not overloading people with information (4) is essential. If they are offered too much information, they will feel overwhelmed and not be able to take it in anyway. You may need to repeat information more than once or even several times. You should look for clues as to how they are managing the shock of the devastating news they have been given and respond accordingly. Giving people enough time to assimilate the fact that their baby has died will also mean that they can begin to ask questions about what happens next. You can ask them if they want you to explain the next steps now or over the next few days if this is appropriate. This is a particular example of when it is helpful for individual patients to have someone with them so that their companion can absorb the information that they cannot take in. With regard to helping people with what happens next, Sands has published a leaflet called *When a baby dies before labour begins*[4] and the hospital where we work has produced one called *What to expect following the death of your baby*.[5] These types of leaflets can be used to back up verbal information.

Support for you (11) is hugely important. You may have to carry on with your normal duties after giving sad news. You need to recognise the impact that telling people sad or bad news has had on you and take appropriate and fitting care of yourself. If possible, negotiate some time away from your normal duties – a chance to have a tea or coffee and a chat with someone.

There are some staff who are at the front line when it comes to giving bad news and we would like to acknowledge them.

SONOGRAPHERS

Sonographers are regularly in the position of discovering either the death of a baby or a baby with an abnormality. It is not uncommon for sonographers to be the first people to know that something is amiss with a pregnancy. This is particularly true in the earlier stages of a baby's development.

Patients often report that they knew something was wrong when they were being scanned because they noticed a change in the sonographer's face or in their demeanour. For the person scanning, setting the scene may mean that every time they scan a pregnant woman they establish a rapport with her and they are specific about the purpose of any particular scan. Despite the fact that women and their families might intellectually know the reason for the nuchal or anomaly scan, this does not mean that they are prepared for something to be wrong. In fact, they are highly unlikely to be prepared, as what we know intellectually bears no relation to what we feel or experience.

When the scan shows that there is something amiss (that the baby has stopped growing or there is an increased nuchal fold, for example), it can be very difficult for both the patient and the sonographer. Hence, there is a need for staff to have practised scenarios that will help them find appropriate ways of dealing with these situations in advance of the real thing.

Research indicates that there are several factors that can help or hinder the way bad news is received.[6] Unsurprisingly, one of the most important factors reported was the empathy of the person giving the news as well as the quality of the information given. This includes what was said as well as whether it was understood by the receiver. The language used when referring to the baby or fetus mattered, too. How the mother refers to her pregnancy should be checked at the outset of a scan. She may say 'baby' or 'fetus' and you should use the same word.

Privacy was highly important to those who took part in the research. The setting where the news is given is worth considering, too, including the physical positions of all those in the room. Is the woman lying down with others standing over her? Does she want to get off the couch and adjust her clothing before a full explanation is given? Is she on her own or does she have her whole family with her including other children?

Negotiating with the woman as to what she wants will require time and it is important that the sonographer does not feel the need to be rushed. This is very difficult when the clinic is busy.

We have said that midwives and doctors are part of a journey that will go on for much longer than their involvement and this is true of a sonographer. Their part in the patient's journey can be good or bad. The skill with which the sonographer imparts difficult news will be remembered by the mother and her family. For example, the senior sonographer where we work is very conscious of this difficult aspect of her role in pregnancy loss and works hard to convey what is likely to be painful information in the most sensitive way possible. One sonographer talked about how she is sometimes identified with the bad or sad news and that she has experienced some patients wanting to avoid her doing another scan as a result. She knows not to take this personally.

It is also important to note that once a mother has received bad news at a scan appointment, it is unlikely that she and her partner will ever be able to take scans for granted again in the future. It is vital the sonographer knows the history of the patient before she comes into their room. If they do not know the patient's history then they are more likely to wonder, for example, why the woman does not want initially to see the ultrasound screen and in this situation the sonographer is in danger of being insensitive. We have known cases of women who have become pregnant again after a loss who are having an early scan to establish the existence of a healthy pregnancy and are asked why they are there. In such a situation, reading the patient's history and the recommendations for her care in a future pregnancy would have provided the sonographer with that information so that the patient would not have experienced being made to feel wrong for having the appointment.

FETAL MEDICINE

One area of caring for pregnant women in which it may be possible to 'set the scene' with regard to giving bad news is in specialist fetal medicine services. The nuchal screening and anomaly scan will highlight that there could be a problem in the baby's development. The patient will then meet specialist staff who will take responsibility for her care. They give the results of blood tests and guide the patient through the options.

In our hospital, there is a fetal medicine lead midwife and a fetal medicine consultant who specialise in working with women who have abnormalities in their pregnancies. They both take a personal interest in caring for and communicating with women and their partners who are faced initially with sad news and then with making difficult decisions regarding the continuation of a pregnancy.

MIDWIVES AND GPs

GPs and antenatal midwives will at some point in their careers be in a position where they are not able to find a baby's heartbeat at a routine antenatal appointment. These staff who are away from the hospital need to arrange for an ultrasound scan for the patient as soon as possible. A midwife already in the hospital needs to be able to do the same.

If you suspect that her baby has died, it is worth preparing the woman for this possibility. You will need to explain why a scan is being offered. It is important to use tact and to try not to alarm her. For example, you can explain that you have not been able to find a heartbeat using a Doppler fetal monitor, that you have some concerns and you want a second opinion to reassure her that all is well with her baby. Do not blame faulty equipment, as the patient will wonder why you are using equipment that does not work! If the woman is on her own, at this point you need to ask her if she would like to get someone to come and be with her. You may need to stay with her or even accompany her to the hospital. If this is impossible, because you are in a GP's surgery or community health centre, you need to ring ahead and confirm with a colleague that they will be ready and waiting for her when she arrives.

LABOUR WARD

Sometimes the labour ward needs to be thought of as akin to the accident and emergency department, as staff on the ward never know what situations they may be dealing with. Therefore, all staff working on the labour ward need to know in advance how to manage setting the scene for giving bad news and then how to help a woman once she has received the devastating information that her baby has died.

Most labour wards have some form of triage suite, where women can be seen, when possible, in order of clinical priority. Women who cannot feel their baby move or who have been sent in by a midwife who has been unable to hear the baby's heartbeat will need to have a scan as soon as possible after arrival, to confirm the diagnosis quickly. It may well be on the labour ward that the news of the baby's demise will be given to the mother and father. Because they have gone to the labour ward, they may already be scared that something is amiss, but they are unlikely to be prepared for the fact that their baby has died or they may be hoping against hope that nothing is wrong.

A quiet room must be available away from the triage suite so that any discussion and ensuing distress can occur in private. This can be a challenge if the room normally used for bereaved women is already occupied, and some thought needs to be given to alternative rooms, preferably away from the sounds of women in labour and crying babies.

SUMMARY

Giving news to patients that will have a painful impact on their lives is hugely important and challenging. However, it is possible to do it well and you can get satisfaction from knowing that you have imparted sad information to parents in a caring and meaningful way. It is no exaggeration to say that they will appreciate this for the rest of their lives.

REFERENCES

1. Kohner N, Leftwich A. *Pregnancy Loss and the Death of a Baby: a training pack for professionals.* Cambridge: National Extension College; 1995.
2. Schott J, Henley A, Kohner N. *Pregnancy Loss and the Death of a Baby: guidelines for professionals.* 3rd ed. London: Sands; 2007.
3. Ross M. *The Conscious Feminine: toolkit.* London: Conscious Feminine Press; 2012.
4. *Sands. When a baby dies before labour begins* [leaflet]. August 2012. Available from Sands, 28 Portland Place, London W1B 1LY.
5. *Lewisham Healthcare NHS Trust. What to expect following the death of your baby.* [leaflet]. March 2011.
6. Alkazaleh F, Thomas M, Grebenyuk J *et al.* What women want: women's preferences of caregiver behaviour when prenatal sonography findings are abnormal. *Ultrasound Obstet Gynecol.* 2004; **23**(1): 56–62.

CHAPTER 4

Initial reactions to grief

INTRODUCTION

A pregnancy loss at any gestation can create grief. It is important to not make assumptions about the level of grief being dependent on the gestation of the baby. This chapter deals with commonly experienced aspects of initial grief, regardless of how early or late in the pregnancy the baby dies.

In our experience, most women who have not experienced a pregnancy loss begin to make plans for the future once they know they are pregnant. They begin to anticipate life with a baby. For example, if other family members or friends are pregnant at the same time they imagine being on maternity leave together and how their babies will be able to play together. We have known people to think about which school their unborn child will attend. It is not unusual for women to know the expected due date, the dates of their scans and their midwife appointments well in advance. These are often marked on their calendar or entered in their diary or mobile phone and when the pregnancy ends they have all these reminders of what is now not happening.

As well as with the actual death of the baby, patients have to come to terms with the loss of the dreams they had about their baby and all that was held in those dreams.

INDIVIDUAL RESPONSES

Individuals, their partners and other family members will have different initial responses to a pregnancy loss. Some will be angry, some will be silent, some will make sense of what has happened through religious or spiritual beliefs, others will cry. You will come across women who seem to be withdrawn and silent and may even appear a bit sullen, or you will have people who are crying either quietly or loudly, though loudly is less common in our experience. There may be family members who do not hold back with their grief (in some cultures it is customary to be extroverted in grief), but in our experience it is rarer for the woman herself to be loud in her distress.

Given the enormity of a baby dying, we are surprised more mothers do not wail with the pain of their loss. It is important to know that however a woman and her family behave, these are their initial ways of coping with the loss. These reactions need to be accepted by all the members of staff they encounter. Accepting patients and their families unconditionally is a prerequisite for looking after them in their grief. It is important that if any of them are angry about something regarding their care that they are listened to. Even if they are wrong, this is not the time to correct them and you need to not get defensive. We know of an incident where security staff were called when a father was angry. This fact stayed with him and for him it added insult to injury. If patients or their relatives are agitated or bordering on becoming aggressive then take those people to a private room and enable them to tell you how they are hurting. Alternatively, you could perhaps clear the room of all unnecessary people, including staff, and give the grieving parents and relatives the time they need. It will help them greatly if you are not frightened by the death of their baby or by any of their reactions. Fear will cause some staff to want to change people's reactions and you may want to make them feel better in some way. This is not possible and it is essential that you do not try. Nothing can make things better; the worst has happened. We do not mean to imply that you are helpless; you are not. Kind, caring and sensitive staff can make an awful situation bearable. Whatever initial reactions people have at the time of being in hospital and in coming to terms with their loss are exactly that: reactions at the beginning of a much longer process of grieving.

We wrote in Chapter 2 about some of the implications of each type of loss, but all types of loss can initially bring about shock. One analogy to use with patients might be that they imagined and experienced themselves going down a particular road with an anticipated destination and then they find that an enormous wall – the death – has suddenly been erected and they have walked straight into it. Most of the time they will not even have known of the possibility of the wall being there, so there is the initial shock of finding themselves in a predicament they had not foreseen. People find this difficult, as they expect that they should have known in advance about something that they could not possibly have known. Then there is the realisation that they have to find a way back from not being able to travel the road they thought they were on. They cannot go back to where they were before they were pregnant. The loss has happened and everyone, to different degrees, will be changed by the loss. Very few situations will have prepared people for coping with the fact that their baby has died and the way they handle it can be likened to any other unexpected event, such as an accident or a disaster, because for many people the end of the pregnancy comes as a complete shock.

The symptoms of emotional and psychological trauma are described below by Robinson *et al.*[1]

> Following a traumatic event, or repeated trauma, people react in different ways, experiencing a wide range of physical and emotional reactions. There is no 'right' or 'wrong' way to think, feel, or respond to trauma, so don't judge your own reactions or those of other people. Your responses are NORMAL reactions to ABNORMAL events. Emotional and psychological symptoms of trauma include:
> - shock, denial or disbelief
> - anger, irritability, mood swings
> - guilt, shame, self-blame
> - feeling sad or hopeless
> - confusion, difficulty concentrating
> - anxiety and fear
> - withdrawing from others
> - feeling disconnected or numb.

These symptoms of trauma are synonymous with the experience of grief. Initially, people need to take in that they have been stopped in their tracks by the fact that their baby has died and that it hurts. They may be left reeling and find it hard to realise what has happened. They will probably only be experiencing shock, denial or disbelief. The other symptoms of grief arise later.

For most patients, this shock will also coincide with the time when they will be required to make decisions regarding the delivery of the baby, how to tell other people, having to make funeral arrangements and so on. To some extent, shock will enable them to make these decisions and carry out some of these arrangements, as they are numb to the enormity of what has happened. It can be useful to think of emotional shock being in some ways similar to physical shock. In physical shock, blood leaves the extremities of the body to go to vital organs to help prolong life. Being in emotional shock means the full impact of what has happened will not necessarily have become real. The normal way of functioning ceases to enable the person to cope with and survive the initial trauma.

People will often look for direction at this time as they are feeling lost. Patients will not be able to think as clearly as they would normally. It is necessary to understand this, as it is the role of the professional to be alongside all those in grief but not to take over. For example, just as with giving bad news, you need to be prepared to give:

➤ the same information as many times as people need it without getting irritable
➤ people time to make up and change their minds
➤ information about all the possibilities regarding the birth and seeing the baby.

In many years of working medically and therapeutically with bereaved parents and their families, we have become very respectful of individual coping mechanisms. Throughout their experience of living, each person will have developed their own responses to life and these will be influenced by the degree of control they have had over what has happened to them. On the whole, people tend to believe they have a lot of control over their own lives. The death of a baby absolutely brings people up against the experience of having no control.

Incidentally, the whole issue of fertility and pregnancy brings people up against the issue of control, though usually the only people who realise this are those who have trouble conceiving or who have had something go wrong. The fact that people get pregnant, stay pregnant and have a healthy baby that survives is actually what is remarkable, not that pregnancy goes wrong. If people have not encountered any difficulty with conceiving or staying pregnant and have a baby who survives labour and lives, they can often think that it was due to themselves. They knew when they were ovulating, they ate the right food and so on; however, it is completely a matter of good fortune that all was well and nothing to do with them personally.

BLAMING THEMSELVES

Given that people think they are much more in control of pregnancy than they actually are, when a pregnancy ends with a death then most people will think that they have done something wrong, which is usually not the case. If there are contributing factors such as smoking, then there are hundreds of examples of women being heavy smokers or even drug users or alcohol abusers who have had healthy full-term babies. This latter fact is very confusing for women who have a pregnancy loss. They wonder why other women who abuse their bodies or their children are able to have a baby and they are not. They become very sensitive to how babies and children are treated.

One of the things that can happen in the initial stages of grieving the death of a baby is that it seems as if other pregnant women and babies are everywhere. There is a heightened awareness of all things connected with pregnancy. Indeed, it is not uncommon for women to report that everything is related to babies, for example, television dramas and advertisements. Even the baby aisle in the supermarket stands out. These all combine to rub in the pain of the loss.

Additionally, women and some partners blame themselves. If they disclose to you that they are taking responsibility for the death of their baby, it is important to make gentle enquiries as to why they are blaming themselves. Many will feel that they must have done something wrong, even if they cannot say specifically what it was. For others, it will be that they did specific things: had a glass of wine, eaten (in ignorance) something that harmed the baby, stressed too much, worked too hard. Retrospectively, they will blame anything that either they thought at the time they were getting away with or gives them a reason why their pregnancy has ended in death. At this time, people are trying to make sense of the death of their baby.

It is helpful to know that the mind likes explanations and finds it very hard if there is no logical reason for something happening. This is another example of our desire to have control and, in the absence of any initial or indeed final explanation for the death, the mind will create ideas about why it happened. Some people are able to reason out that these thoughts are incorrect but others feel tormented. It feels that almost any explanation is better than none. People do not want to be at fault – indeed, it is something they dread – however, what it would mean is that there is a rational reason to explain their loss and that they have something to avoid the next time they are pregnant.

THE EARLY DAYS OF GRIEF

The first few days or weeks of loss are taken up with the actual loss: for example, with a miscarriage, there is the operation to remove retained products and with a stillbirth there is giving birth. Then there are other things to be done: registering the baby, visiting the baby in the mortuary or funeral home, making funeral arrangements and the funeral itself. These things are all to do with the actual death of the baby and to some extent keep people busy. At this time, for many bereaved parents there are often a lot of people around. Family members and friends are very concerned and they want to comfort and console.

There is an intensity of experience at this time and often it is only when this ends that the other aspects of emotional and psychological symptoms of grief described earlier begin to show. What people begin to realise is that as well as the pain of the death itself, they have to grieve for the loss of their baby and all of its implications. These other aspects of grief and mourning will be explored further on.

SUMMARY

The initial reactions to grief are profoundly demanding. All those involved in the loss are vulnerable and they need to be cared for by kind, competent and empathic staff who can show them their humanity.

REFERENCE

1. Robinson L, Smith M, Segal J. Healing emotional and psychological trauma. Updated June 2012. Available at: www.helpguide.org/mental/emotional_psychological_trauma.htm (accessed 26 August 2012).

CHAPTER 5

Patient-centred care

INTRODUCTION

This chapter deals with the basic elements of care that you need to make 'the unbearable bearable' when looking after women and their families who are managing the death of their baby.

Patient-centred care has many definitions, but a well-accepted one is offered by the Institute of Medicine and quoted by the King's Fund:[1]

> [P]roviding care that is respectful of and responsive to individual patient preferences, needs, and values and ensuring that patient values guide all clinical decisions. In today's NHS [National Health Service] it has come to mean putting the patient and their experience at the heart of quality improvement. Patient-centred care is one aspect of health care quality, as important as care being safe, clinically effective, timely and equitable.

Patient-centred care is multidimensional; it encompasses all aspects of how services are delivered to patients. The Institute of Medicine[1] offers this list:

➤ compassion, empathy and responsiveness to needs, values and expressed preferences
➤ emotional support, relieving fear and anxiety
➤ coordination and integration
➤ physical comfort
➤ involvement of family and friends
➤ information, communication and education.

This list is in a different order from the original, to relate better to caring for bereaved women.

Some of these aspects stand out when thinking about the immediate care needed for patients, partners and families around the time of the death and others need to be enshrined permanently into policies. They also apply to the support that staff need to enable them to do their jobs effectively.

In this chapter, we consider this list in relation to patients, partners and their families.

COMPASSION, EMPATHY AND RESPONSIVENESS TO NEEDS, VALUES AND EXPRESSED PREFERENCES

It is absolutely essential that these three qualities be at the forefront of care for women giving birth to their baby who has died. It is important to understand that compassion and empathy are not the same as feeling sorry for someone or pitying them. The *Free Dictionary* definition of 'compassion' indicates that it is synonymous with an 'awareness of the suffering of another coupled with a wish to relieve it'.[2] You cannot change what has happened, but you can make an important contribution to the experiences women and their families have surrounding the death of their baby and the loss of all the dreams associated with the baby. You need to be kind, caring and not overwhelmed by how difficult you might be finding the event.

Remember that just being there can make a difference. You need to be open to the myriad ways in which women and their family members respond to their loss. Your patient may want to talk. Alternatively, she may not want to talk; she may want to turn her face to the pillow and pretend to sleep. You may feel that you are not able to engage with her at all, but it is likely that just knowing you are there for her will mean something to her and her family.

Being there is not passive. It does not mean avoiding what is happening; it means being sensitive to the needs of your patient. It also does not mean hiding behind the task of writing your notes when the patient appears not to need you. You may think 'it is okay; she doesn't seem to need me at the moment, so I'll get on with my notes'. The patient may think afterwards 'all she did was write her notes'. The way to avoid any possibility of this type of misunderstanding is to say something like 'I'm here for you; I'll be here writing some notes, let me know if there is anything specific you need. I'm here to make sure you're as okay as you can be.'

Being able to be responsive to the needs, values and preferences, both expressed and unexpressed, of the patient requires you to have the ability to communicate. We cannot emphasise enough the importance of communication and we acknowledge that it is demanding. You will need to use all your senses to understand what is needed. Almost moment by moment you have to be ready to anticipate your patient's and her family's needs. Patients may require you to tell them what options they have regarding their care and the care of their baby. Most women will not have been in these circumstances before, and even if they have it does not mean that they know exactly what they want or what to do. For example, we know of one woman who was suffering her third mid-trimester loss, who, when she started to pass clots, was told by a nurse 'you've been through this before, you know what to do' and was then left to cope on her own. She was rightly furious about this lack of care. She felt abandoned at a time when she was, arguably, even more vulnerable because of her previous losses.

When caring for a woman who is giving birth to her baby who has died, it behoves you to be very clear within yourself about being open-minded to all sorts of possibilities regarding what patients might need. It may help you to adopt an attitude of 'Why not?' rather than 'Why?' or 'This is not what people normally want.' For a woman whose baby is not going to be born alive, nothing is normal. Women and their families have so little time to be with their baby. The time following the birth is so precious. Being able to visit their baby subsequently in the mortuary is hugely important to some, but their baby will not be the same as she was immediately after birth and in the hours following. If someone wants to do something you have not experienced anyone else doing, you can support them unless it will cause harm to the patient.

One woman who did not see her baby naked wished someone had suggested it or had asked her if she wanted to do so. Retrospectively, she did not know if she would have wanted to look at her naked daughter, but she regretted the fact that no one had mentioned it as a possibility. The reason she became aware of what she had potentially missed as another opportunity to relate to her daughter was that she heard from other women in the local support group (Sands – for those who have had a stillbirth or neonatal death) describing what they had done. She will never have that opportunity again.

It is also necessary to be prepared for patients not being ready or wanting to do what is perceived as good practice. For example, a woman whose daughter died soon after birth objected strongly to being told she should dress her baby as it would help her. For her it was not something she wanted to do at that time. There are no 'shoulds' in relation to patients and how they manage the death of their baby, so you must never impose them. Instead, you can make suggestions or explain what you know other women in their situation have done.

EMOTIONAL SUPPORT

It is crucial that caregivers are prepared for any, all kinds of, or no obvious emotional response to the death of a baby. You must allow for the fact that different members of the same family will have different ways of expressing their emotions. The Child Bereavement Charity[3] has a helpful leaflet called *Women, men and grief* that illustrates the different ways men and women grieve.

Often when people are given the news that their baby has died, they will go into emotional shock: this may translate into a form of numbness, which can last for hours, days or even weeks. Initially, the death may seem unreal. Within psychological circles, a well-known expression is 'under stress we regress'. This saying means that when we are unable to control life or life events (stress), we regress to an earlier, or even our earliest, way of dealing with control issues. Therefore, you will meet patients and their supporters who express helplessness, anger, fury, blame, despair, anxiety and so forth. It is not your job to *react* to whatever emotion is or is not being expressed. It is your job to *respond* to these reactions, as this will mean that you are more likely to continue to be kind and understanding. Let us explain what we mean by the difference between 'reaction' and 'response'. It is almost impossible not to have a reaction to a situation or an event; reactions tend to be instantaneous. In contrast, responses tend to be more thought out and give you and any other person more room to move. For example, if someone is rude to you, your reaction may lead you to want to be rude back, to complain loudly or to do something else; however, your response will include the ability to think about the consequences of any reaction.

Some staff find it very upsetting when women cry and scream because of the extent of their loss, whilst others see this sort of noisy reaction as entirely appropriate. Conversely, others find a patient who remains completely silent very unnerving. They may feel they have to try to fill the silence by saying something and often they may end up saying the wrong thing. It is important that you learn which reactions to grief you find challenging and which you personally find more natural and understandable.

Reactions are not right or wrong; they are natural to the women involved and also to the staff. Whilst women and their families dealing with their grief cannot avoid reacting, staff need to be able to respond to the women rather than letting their own emotional reactions to expressions of grief interfere with their care.

We know of a woman who, having lost a baby as a result of meconium aspiration, went to the ward reception area to ask for painkillers. The midwife, who did not know her case (but the patient would have expected that she did and she was right in having that expectation), said 'Is being in pain what's making you look so miserable?' and the woman replied that the reason she looked miserable was because her baby had died. This lack of awareness and the midwife reacting to the way a patient looked caused a great deal of distress for an already grieving mother, and could so easily have been avoided. It is example of 'if only': if only the midwife had simply given her some painkillers or had been aware of the issues for patients on her ward then this situation would not have arisen. As it was, a crass reaction by someone the patient was expecting to care added insult to injury and will never be forgotten.

You have to be kind and patient. It will be useful to you if you understand that you are involved in a small part of a much longer journey and that how you are during your part in accompanying the patient and her family along the way will have either a positive or negative impact.

RELIEVING FEAR AND ANXIETY
First, you need to find out if patients, their partners and families are feeling afraid and anxious. By asking those involved if they are fearful and anxious, you will be better able to respond to their needs rather than if you assume you know already. By allowing patients and their families to talk about what they are frightened of, you will be helping by listening and, where appropriate, trying to alleviate their fears. You can, for example, explain the process of birth and what they can expect once their baby is born. You can talk normally and naturally to the parents about the baby they were expecting and who they are now never going to have.

It is essential that you do not project your fear and anxiety on to them. If you find that you are scared or apprehensive then you need to get support from your colleagues so that you have the chance to examine what it is that frightens you. This is of course best done before you start caring for a bereaved family.

COORDINATION AND INTEGRATION
The lack of coordination between staff within the hospital, as well as with those who work in the community, is one of the reasons women complain about their treatment. This lack of coordination can leave women and their

families feeling uncared for. You need to ensure that all the people involved in the mother's care are kept informed about what has happened, and that, regardless of who is looking after her, the quality of her care is paramount. Any transfer of care should be as seamless as possible. Handovers should include how you have looked after the patient and her family, what their current status is, both emotional and physical, and what their needs are, as well as reporting the bare facts. All other colleagues, such as morticians, community midwives, GPs and other necessary specialists, need to know what has happened. This way, everyone is aware not only of the loss, but also of the individual patient's needs. We have heard too many times how a community midwife has turned up at a patient's home without being informed that they are visiting a bereaved family, not a family with a live born baby.

PHYSICAL COMFORT

When we are hurting emotionally, physical pain can be more intense and when we are hurting physically, emotional pain can be worse. When you are involved in examining a woman, it can be immensely helpful to know that her capacity to cope with or endure any kind of physical pain may well be greatly reduced. Much of this will be covered in Chapter 7, 'Labour and delivery', but we would like to mention some points relevant to the initial diagnosis of a pregnancy loss.

It is vital that in every department within the hospital in which bereaved parents will be managed, their physical comfort as well as their emotional and mental well-being have been considered. These areas can include the emergency department, the antenatal clinic, the early pregnancy unit, the labour ward and the gynaecology ward. All of these areas need to have the facility to allow the mother's partner or her chosen companion to stay with her for the duration of her care. It means being flexible and enabling her partner (as well as herself) to be made as physically comfortable as possible, including during any overnight stay.

Another example would be that if a woman is waiting for a scan to confirm the death of her baby, consideration has been given to where she will wait, how she will be informed, who is with her, what her needs are and where she goes after the scan. It is not appropriate for her to be with other women in an antenatal waiting room. If she is left in a quiet room to await another member of staff, she should be told how long this might take, and that someone will check on her regularly and keep her informed as to what is happening. It also means ensuring that she and those with her are given the time they need to understand what has happened. You may need to ask a colleague to take over your other duties whilst you attend to the needs of the bereaved mother and her family.

INVOLVEMENT OF FAMILY AND FRIENDS

As we said earlier, whilst coming to terms with the death of a baby, for the grieving family you are a small but essential part of their journey. Family and friends are hopefully going to be there for a much longer time. The mother and her partner (if she has one) must be at the heart of deciding whom they want to be informed, involved and present. Sometimes individuals or couples do not want anyone else to be present, whilst others want a select few or many people to participate in this part of their bereavement.

Just as you can be a guide in relation to helping a mother and her family decide on what is right for them in terms of seeing and holding their baby and so forth, you can help bereaved patients by knowing what is possible in the widest sense. To do this, you must not have any preconceived ideas about what is or not right for any one person or family. For example, one woman, after inquiring whether her other children should see the baby, was told by a midwife that she did not think it would be helpful. It is necessary to understand that your opinion is not relevant in these situations, even though it is tempting to think that it is. Giving your own personal opinion is exactly that and your opinion is only relevant to you. Furthermore, if you were in the situation of your patient, you might not even have the same opinion as you have on her behalf.

Understanding that when someone asks a question there is often a statement behind the question can help you at these times. It is much better for the patient and for yourself if you can help elucidate the statement rather than answer a direct question. What the patient needs is for you to help her to come to her own conclusion; what she does not need is your opinion. So, in relation to being asked the question as to whether it would be helpful for her other children to see the baby, the mother's statement might have been something like 'I don't know whether to let my other children see their baby brother.' In this case, the midwife could have helped the mother explore what her thoughts were regarding the pros and cons of the children meeting their brother. That way she would have arrived at the complexities that the mother was considering. She would have helped the mother by enabling her to express her thoughts or worries and this would probably have led to her making the right decision for her in respect of her family.

Many families will not question the idea of their other children seeing the baby. These families will have the baby's siblings hold and cuddle the baby and will take photographs of them with the baby. Others will want to protect their children from any experience of the baby's death. As a healthcare professional, your job is to help those who know what they want to achieve this. For those who do not know what they want, you can help them by exploring all the options with them. This requires you to have an open mind and an ability to accept whatever people choose once they have been given the choices.

INFORMATION, COMMUNICATION AND EDUCATION

Information and communication need to be at the heart of the care offered to women, their partners and families. Information is vital for people, particularly if they are in shock. It can ease their anxiety. For most women, their baby dying will not have been what they expected. Even when the death of a baby is anticipated, it does not mean it is expected. It is vitally important that they are told what to expect once the diagnosis of a death or fatal illness has been given. Knowing what to anticipate when the unexpected has happened is essential. It will help the patient and her family feel more secure and is likely to make the patient feel understood, cared for and somewhat prepared for what happens next.

Any information given has to be in accordance with the patient's needs. It is often appropriate that spoken information is backed up with leaflets, such as those from ARC, Sands, the Miscarriage Association and patient-information leaflets from your own hospital. These can give vital help in guiding patients through the process of the hospital experience and beyond.

You need to make sure that the correct leaflets are given at the right time. For example, it is no good giving someone a leaflet about caring for their baby at the time of birth once they have gone home and it is not useful to give a funeral arrangements booklet before birth unless this has been specifically requested.

As we have emphasised, good communication is vital to patient-centred care. Communication and the giving of information is a two-way process. It is not just your job to tell people what they need to know from the organisation's viewpoint; you also need to get to know your patient and other relevant family members and to establish a rapport with them, so that you can communicate well. People who are scared or hurting may find it hard to take in what is being said unless it is what they want to hear, so it will be necessary to understand what they are feeling and take this into account when you are talking to them.

Communication is not just about giving patients information, facts or figures. Communication includes:

➤ finding out what patients are expecting
➤ helping them to understand the appropriateness of these expectations
➤ actively listening to what you are being told
➤ actively listening to what is not being said and exploring this
➤ watching for and responding to the way that what you are saying is being received
➤ establishing that what you are saying is being understood appropriately (i.e. that you are going at the patient's pace)
➤ meaning what you say, not setting up false expectations for yourself or for patients; for example, if you promise to be in touch with people, be clear about when you will contact them, and make sure that you do contact them when you have said you will
➤ using words and explanations that are patient-centred and not medical jargon
➤ allowing time for information to be understood and processed
➤ allowing time for questions and for information to be repeated as required
➤ giving space for emotional reactions and being non-judgemental about these.

Every patient and the members of her family need an individual response to their unique experience. They have different needs, wants and desires. Additionally, you are also dealing with any previous involvement they had regarding their own or other's medical treatment. For example, some people view the hospital negatively or positively, which might be associated in the former case with someone's father dying or in the latter by someone being cured during their stay.

Remember, too, that often it is the very small details that patients will hold on to, the good or the bad. As well as checking the expectations that the woman and her relatives have, you need to be aware of any expectations you may inadvertently be setting up, particularly in the area of being specific. For example, do not say that you will be back in a minute. No one would expect that you really would be back in 1 minute, but if you are not back in 10 minutes then they may begin to wonder. If you give a specific time and are unable to fulfil that, go and tell the patient that they are not forgotten. One of the things that can happen when people are grieving is that their ability to tolerate waiting may be diminished. When their baby dies, people are bearing the unbearable; you must not be party to causing them more anxiety and distress on top of that excruciating pain.

SUMMARY

This chapter is about putting the care of the patient and her needs, together with those of her loved ones, at the forefront of any service. These needs are of paramount importance and require that members of staff work towards meeting them appropriately, with kindness and understanding. It does not mean having to know everything in advance, as each individual and family are unique. It does mean that the organisation supports its staff to enable them to put patient-centred care at the heart of their service.

REFERENCES

1. www.kingsfund.org.uk/topics/patientcentred_care/ (accessed 29 August 2012).
2. www.thefreedictionary.com/compassion (accessed 29 August 2012).
3. Thomas J, Samuel J. Women, men and grief (Child Bereavement Charity information sheet). Available at: www.childbereavement.org.uk

CHAPTER 6

Support for staff

INTRODUCTION

This chapter is about staff and their needs in relation to pregnancy loss. Whilst instinctive supportive words and gestures cannot be taught, there are some basic principles that might be useful to consider when dealing with the shock and sense of loss that attends perinatal death. Most of the requirements for patient-centred care can be employed in thinking about supporting staff and we have used these requirements to elucidate our ideas regarding staff support.

Almost all of the principles and values deemed necessary for patient-centred care apply to supporting staff. We would argue that these attributes are important all of the time in providing care within the National Health Service, which might then make looking after women who are dealing with the death of their baby less formidable. In our experience, it is necessary to accept that some staff will naturally be better than others at looking after women who are in the unfortunate position of having a baby die. For many, the giving of support in times of trouble is natural and instinctive. It feels clumsy and awkward for others, like trying to pronounce unfamiliar words or forcing limbs into uncomfortable positions.

It is highly likely that some members of staff will have experienced a pregnancy loss themselves and this may make them better at supporting patients whose babies die or else make them less able to provide the care needed. These sensitive personal circumstances need to be acknowledged and respected. For this to happen, there needs to be a pre-existing and permanent atmosphere of trust and safety between the management and all members of staff in the maternity unit.

Hospitals and other agencies need to decide whether it is better to have the expectation that all staff will be required to provide a service to those women and their families or whether there will be nominated or even dedicated staff who will take on that role. If all of the staff are required to be able to provide a service, there is the risk that bereaved mothers will be looked after by dis-interested or frightened midwives or doctors who will not be able to care for them and their relatives as required.

Whatever the policy regarding staffing, it is essential that regular training and support for staff working with pregnancy loss be built into the system. Individual staff should not have to be responsible for having to find their own support.

STAFF-CENTRED DELIVERY OF CARE

We have used the same list[1] as in the previous chapter:
➤ information, communication and education
➤ compassion, empathy and responsiveness to needs, values and expressed preferences
➤ emotional support, relieving fear and anxiety
➤ coordination and integration
➤ physical comfort
➤ involvement of family and friends.

The order of this list has been changed from the original to make it more appropriate for staff support.

Staff groups and individual staff members require compassion, empathy and responsiveness to needs, values and expressed preferences. For example, there will be staff from cultures where terminations will be against the law or at odds with their religious belief who might have their own objections to being present for a feticide or a therapeutic termination. Alternatively, there may be staff who do not object but who will be inexperienced in the procedures and will need extra training and support.

The way that compassion, empathy and responsiveness to needs, values and expressed preferences is offered will differ from how they are given to the patient, as it less likely that they can be offered 'in the moment'. However, there may be times when senior staff will need to recognise that a particular staff member is not in a fit state to care for a bereaved mother. Being on a busy and demanding labour ward may lead managers to feel annoyed with staff who are having difficulty, but it is important to adopt an attitude of understanding and care. Incidentally, if this kind of management exists, it is probable that it will be reflected in the care offered to all patients, regardless of whether there is a pregnancy loss.

Information, communication and education are vital to enable staff to do their job properly and responsibly. Complaints, when broken down to the basic errors, often indicate that a lack of communication and information was central to the complaint. Staff need to know how to access policies and procedures so that they are *au fait* with what information they require. They need guidelines on how to provide the practical aspects of caring and they need a structure that enables them to include the emotional side of caring.

Communication between different departments is basic and a central aspect of care. It is essential that staff do not limit their thinking to their own area of work. Forethought is necessary and when it is present patients will not be aware of it. If it is not present, patients will definitely be aware and are likely to suffer as a result. An example of this kind of lack of forethought is putting a woman whose baby is in the neonatal unit and likely to die, in a room on the postnatal ward with women who have their babies with them. Having no consideration for a patient's reality can be really upsetting and lead to her feeling uncared for. In turn, she may then become suspicious of other staff. If situations like this are not understood and handled correctly then they can lead to more injury as staff turn against a 'difficult' patient.

> Tell me and I will forget;
> Show me and I may remember;
> Involve me and I will understand.
> *Chinese Proverb*

INFORMATION, COMMUNICATION AND EDUCATION

These requirements are the touchstone for staff caring for women with a pregnancy loss. We would also add respect as a vital ingredient in supporting staff. These qualities need to be integral to the workplace. Management will need to offer training and supervision that is ongoing and appropriate to the needs of the individuals involved in service provision around pregnancy loss. Any death may remind individuals of their own experiences of loss and it is essential that staff are able to separate themselves from their own feelings so they can be truly present for the patient. If workers are unable to divorce themselves from their own experience of grief then they need to know that there are senior members of staff with whom they can discuss these matters and know that they will be understood. Senior staff may need to make an immediate decision to remove the midwife or doctor from the situation or, in the longer term, they may need to support that staff member to have bereavement counselling.

Most perinatal loss patients, especially those who have suffered a stillbirth or neonatal death or who have had any complications, need to be seen and managed by experienced members of staff. It is unfair to all concerned to expect junior staff to deal with the clinical and emotional fallout of a stillbirth or neonatal death without senior support. Some trusts have policies in place to ensure senior involvement; for example, there may be in-house rules about the seniority required to discuss and sign a consent form for a PM examination of the baby. Nevertheless, these situations present a valuable opportunity to teach by example as long as they are sensitively handled.

We know that many nurses, midwives and doctors want to learn how to improve their skills and their ability to care and they need regular opportunities to do so. They want to know what to say, how to say it and what to do to help a patient who is grieving. Learning is important, as it helps people gain skills and knowledge and, perhaps more importantly in this challenging area, to become confident in learning how to be and what to do.

If you are the senior midwife allocated to look after a woman being induced because of a perinatal death, explain to her that you have a student midwife working with you for that week and ask if it would be all right for the student to accompany you. Many patients have actually reported that the student midwife was extremely caring and helpful to them. This may be because the student has no other defined role and is free to give emotional support.

If you are the senior obstetrician covering the labour ward on the day that a stillborn baby is delivered, when you go into the patient's room you can, if it feels appropriate, gently ask if you may bring in a junior colleague or a student. Your junior colleague can accompany you and learn about what happens in perinatal loss cases in a protected way. It is good manners to introduce yourself and your colleague ('This is Charlie, he's a student on my team and he's working with me today . . .'). Whilst your patient may not be doing much talking and may not visibly react, she may remember things that you say to her with great clarity. Your junior colleague does not need to say anything but can watch the interaction between you and the mother.

This sort of exposure can help to defuse the fear some juniors may have about approaching bereaved patients. Those who have an innate sense of how to behave will mirror your behaviour and find that they are comfortable even in such a potentially distressing situation. One of my (Ruth's) former students came with me to see a woman whose dead baby boy had been born earlier that morning. I crouched by the bed to talk to her so as not to be towering over her whilst she cradled her son in her arms. I realised that the student was crouching too, to be on the same level as the two of us. I had not told him to do this; he did it instinctively. Later on, he went back to talk to her on his own. When I saw the mother for a follow-up appointment some weeks later, she mentioned the student by name and told me what a comfort it had been to be able to talk to someone who was so naturally kind and sympathetic.

Another way of gaining confidence and learning with regard to pregnancy loss is enabling staff to have regular opportunities to discuss their experiences of dealing with baby death. We advocate that this is not just when they have been directly involved in a death. Staff need to be able to learn from one another; they need to ask difficult questions of themselves and each other in a non-judgemental atmosphere.

Individual members of staff who have looked after a woman and her family may well need an opportunity to talk to their supervisor or mentor very soon after they have finished their shift and we think that it is the senior member of staff who holds the responsibility for ensuring this happens. Support should not be left to the individual concerned. This is where the model of supervision used in the counselling profession can be a useful one to adopt. In this discipline, supervision and support are not seen as something only to be offered when someone is not coping but as a regular commitment to the development and understanding of the role the counsellor plays.

It is perhaps unrealistic to expect that individual weekly or fortnightly supervision can be offered to medical staff. However, we would recommend that individuals who have been involved in caring for a woman whose baby has died are contacted by a senior staff member within a short space of time following the event and are given care and an opportunity to have a debriefing meeting. This is beneficial not just because it will help if the midwife or doctor has found it a difficult task but also to encourage those who have an aptitude for caring in sensitive situations. We believe that people should be given support when things are going well as much as when they are struggling. We are talking about fostering an atmosphere of trust, appreciation and respect as a given. This will help when difficult circumstances arise.

Often, it is only when a birth has been particularly difficult that it is recognised that staff need support. We would argue that there needs to be a forum for reflection and learning that is available to staff even when things have gone well. Very rarely in our experience do staff get regular credit for good work from within the organisation, which adds to their feelings of frustration and can leave them resentful when they feel they are blamed for errors.

Communication is not automatic: there is a saying that most dialogues are monologues, with each person just waiting to say their piece rather than having the ability to respond to the other person. Therefore, the art of communication needs to be understood and appreciated. Staff need opportunities to practise what real communication is before they look after women. Throughout the book, we give examples of good communication when dealing with patients and we think it is equally important that senior staff apply these principles to their dealings with staff as well as offering them training.

COMPASSION, EMPATHY AND RESPONSIVENESS TO NEEDS, VALUES AND EXPRESSED PREFERENCES

Patient-centred care is a necessity in our work and we would like to propose that the same principle applies when supporting staff who care for women with a pregnancy loss. Patients want to feel that they are individuals and that they are not just another number. It is the same for staff.

It may be helpful to reflect on whether it is possible for a staff member within your organisation to express a preference for not looking after patients who are giving birth to a dead baby. If not, why not? We have found that when staff are reluctant to care, this is exactly what happens: their care comes across as reluctant and everyone suffers as a result, including the hospital legal department.

Just as patients need to know they are cared for, so do staff. This does not mean that staff should not be expected to carry out their job professionally and responsibly; however, everyone can blossom and flourish in an atmosphere where good practice is rewarded and where individual efforts are acknowledged. Many people only find out how important they are to their workplace when they read the positive comments written on their leaving cards. We think this is a pity.

EMOTIONAL SUPPORT, RELIEVING FEAR AND ANXIETY

It can be daunting looking after women and their families during and after a pregnancy loss. Members of staff need opportunities to be able to explore their emotional response to death, grieving and bereavement in relation to pregnancy and receive emotional support in return. Support is about helping staff as they go along. It can be explicit or tacit. It is also important that staff have help with being part of, but separate from, all the drama that necessarily surrounds the death of a baby.

It is not unusual for caregivers to feel fear and anxiety initially at the thought of caring for people who are in the throes of coming to terms with their baby's death. However, if they are given the right kind of help to understand that they have a valid and valuable role to play, then their fear and anxiety can be greatly reduced.

Supporting means helping people come to terms with what their experience has been, as their experiences may have been difficult and dramatic. This can be especially true if the baby dies at the time of delivery. Individual and group debriefs can be helpful. You need a neutral facilitator who can engender a non-judgemental atmosphere in which staff can talk openly and honestly about their actions, feelings and thoughts regarding the situation they have participated in. As we have said previously, staff need encouragement when they are doing well and we want to emphasise that staff also need support when they are feeling demoralised, hopeless, frustrated or dreadful.

COORDINATION AND INTEGRATION

The necessity of looking after women and their families who have a baby die is going to be part of any maternity service. It is not separate from the rest of what is on offer; the care, attention to detail and tenderness required when women are bereaved must be an integrated part of the whole service. If the care given to the majority of women who have happy experiences of live births is good and the hospital has developed a positive reputation, there is no reason why it cannot have the same for looking after bereaved mothers and fathers.

Coordination is an indispensable part of, and central to, good care. Individual caregivers need to communicate with others, including all the professionals who have dealings with the mother and her family. This kind of coordination and integration may require consideration of shift patterns, changing them when necessary to ensure continuity of care and ensuring that handovers are not perfunctory but include detailed information of 'who' the patient is, including an adequate personal history and relevant facts regarding her cultural beliefs.

It also means having a system where the labour ward coordinator is supernumerary and that individual midwives and doctors have immediate access to their supervisors and to support in any crisis. Any recriminations can come later. Clear and concise instructions need to be available to staff so that they can know what to do. All necessary information should be readily available on the ward. Where we work, there is a midwives' checklist that takes staff through each step of providing support for patients and gives details of the paperwork required. Staff should also know how to gain access to policies and procedures that are stored electronically.

PHYSICAL COMFORT

It should be ensured that staff have safe places to 'retire' to whilst they are managing their experience of looking after patients. This may also mean that they need reassurance, which can be given through a hug, an arm around the shoulder or a hand held. As with patients, it is important that this is done with the member of staff's consent. Each member of staff is an individual and each will have their own coping mechanisms. These coping mechanisms need to be respected as long as they are not detrimental to the individual or their work. As with patients, nothing should be done without their consent and it is perfectly okay to ask colleagues what they need when you see them.

The very first in-house training provided for midwives regarding pregnancy loss at our unit was interesting in that it raised a request from staff that managers actually make them cups of tea when they have experienced a traumatic death or the delivery of a dead baby. This seemed to be an expression of wanting to be looked after and given care and appreciation in a very obvious and demonstrable way.

INVOLVEMENT OF FAMILY AND FRIENDS

Even if the support from the workplace is exemplary, it is still likely that staff will need the understanding and cooperation of their family and friends. They often know the individual better than anyone else.

However, although we may have support from family and friends, as caregivers we also need to know how to look after ourselves following difficult experiences at work. We need to have a good work–life balance. It is not only helpful but also responsible to look after ourselves following a shift in which we have been involved in a baby's death, especially in the immediate aftermath. It is good practice to complete all notes before leaving work; this is not only good practice on a personal level but also essential in relation to any clinical inquiry. In this way, as individuals we can consciously try to leave work behind us when we leave at the end of the shift.

Conscientious people often feel they cannot just leave, but it is essential that you know your limits and give yourself permission to go home. This can be a difficult decision to make. We have known bereaved parents express enormous gratitude that the midwife or doctor who was initially looking after them stayed on long after their shift had finished because they cared. This kind of commitment needs to be appreciated and any staff working overtime must have their time back. Having an emotional response to working with any patient is not a sign of weakness. It can be the absolute opposite and an indication that the individual staff member cares. Caring is a fundamental requirement for women and their families. Any dilemma of this nature is helped enormously by the individual knowing that there are others within the workplace who will carry on caring and taking appropriate responsibility. The ability to be able to know this will depend on the degree of trust and camaraderie that exists in any unit.

You need to have good food to eat for nourishment. You need the ability to deal with any sleep disturbance in a healthy way. A routine that involves meditation or relaxation can help you sleep without disturbing thoughts waking you up. If this does occur, it is sometimes very helpful to write down all the thoughts, feelings, fears or anxieties that are keeping you awake, without censoring yourself. This can leave your brain and your mind clear enough to enable restful sleep. The writing can then be used in the daytime to inform you of any unfinished business. It is not unusual for people to be awake during the night and then worry about not getting enough sleep, but the thoughts that appear during this time are often very creative and informative. They can tell you, for example, if you are angry with colleagues, the system or even the patient. It may well be important to act on information gained in this way, either for your own sake or for the sake of others in similar situations, by giving feedback to appropriate colleagues. This kind of care is really worth cultivating, but it is crucial that it is not a substitute for the professional and personal care that staff have a right to expect from their workplace.

SUMMARY

This chapter emphasises that the care patients receive is dependent on the quality of the support provided for staff. If the workplace values and motivates individual staff members to be the best possible professionals they can be, then patients will benefit hugely. If this fostering of good relationships is absent then the care patients receive will be down to single workers who will quickly burn out and probably leave.

REFERENCE
1. www.kingsfund.org.uk/topics/patientcentred_care/ (accessed 29 August 2012).

CHAPTER 7

Labour and delivery

This chapter discusses what staff should expect regarding labour and delivery at different gestations. We give ideas about how to help patients to cope and how staff can learn to cope themselves.

FIRST TRIMESTER MISCARRIAGES

First trimester miscarriages either happen spontaneously or are delayed or missed and may have to be removed by evacuation of the uterus (ERPC). Early miscarriages of this sort end without labour and delivery, but women will often talk about 'losing the baby'. When talking to women about early losses, it is important to take your cue from them and to use the language that they use rather than trying to impose your own different vocabulary.

SECOND TRIMESTER MISCARRIAGE AND TERMINATION

From 13 weeks' gestation, the options for ending a pregnancy are an ERPC, using suction if there has been a delayed miscarriage; a dilatation and evacuation (D&E); or an induced miscarriage. An ERPC or a suction TOP, if the fetal parts are small enough for this to be appropriate, will usually be carried out under general anaesthesia. It is helpful to have suction curettes available that are wider than the usual maximum of 12 mm (say, 14 mm and 16 mm) and wider-bore suction tubing, as this makes the procedure quicker. The patient may want to be given the products of conception after any laboratory analysis has been carried out, perhaps so that she can bury them in her garden, for example, and enquiries must be made about this before the procedure is undertaken. Otherwise, unless there are recognisable fetal parts in the products, the remains will be examined by the laboratory staff and then disposed of in whichever manner the hospital has arranged.

A D&E can be carried out by a suitably experienced obstetrician up to about 16 weeks' gestation or even further. It involves removing the pregnancy piecemeal whilst the patient is anaesthetised. The remains will not be suitable for viewing or photographs afterwards. There is a significant risk of uterine perforation and damage to other organs. Watching a D&E can be extremely distressing for the staff in the operating theatre, as they will be able to recognise the pieces of the baby being removed and collected by the surgeon; this is counterbalanced by the woman undergoing the operation being oblivious to the proceedings.

An induced miscarriage is used to end a second trimester pregnancy, especially after 16 weeks in cases where there is a fetal abnormality, as the baby will be delivered intact and a PM can be performed. Contractions will be induced using misoprostol 100 mcg every 6 hours. The process is the same regardless of whether the baby is alive or dead, except that if he is alive before the proceeding begins, it will be a termination and Certificate A will have been signed by two doctors first. If the gestation is at 20 weeks or more, feticide should be carried out first to prevent the baby being born alive.

Some staff will have a conscientious objection to termination and this must be respected. The midwife in charge must be aware of any objections when allocating midwives to look after women at the beginning of a shift. That said, all staff have a duty of care when required, so if a woman who has had a medical termination has a haemorrhage, you cannot refuse to help her, even if you disagreed with the termination.

The placenta is often retained after a mid-trimester loss, so it is wise to discuss manual removal of the placenta with the patient at the start of the process and warn her that this might be necessary. It may also be worth obtaining formal consent for manual removal before the induction begins, rather than trying to do it after the delivery when the woman is likely to be more upset and distracted.

From 20 weeks' gestation, women will make breast milk following delivery, so cabergoline 1 mg must be prescribed and given to women soon after they have delivered to prevent this. Failure to do this can be very distressing. For them to have milk oozing from their breasts whilst coming to terms with the death of their baby can cause confusion and pain.

LATER SECOND AND THIRD TRIMESTER LOSSES

The remainder of this chapter deals with later losses, and with the various aspects of preparation for labour, induction, the labour itself, the delivery and its aftermath.

IUFD: diagnosis

At any time in their pregnancy from about 26 weeks onwards, women may come to the maternity unit saying that they have stopped feeling their baby moving. If a woman presents with reduced or absent fetal movements, and a fetal heart is not audible with a Doppler fetal monitor, she must have a scan to determine whether the baby has died. All senior and middle-grade obstetric staff will be able to scan to check for a beating fetal heart, and there must be a functioning ultrasound machine available for use on the labour ward so that this can be done without delay. Most units will have a policy requiring a second opinion in such cases, even if the diagnosis is obvious from the first scan. The second opinion will usually be supplied by the consultant obstetrician on call, but may in some circumstances be requested from a sonographer. By arranging a second scan, you are seeking to confirm the diagnosis of fetal death: the parents may interpret the second scan as a chance that their baby is still alive, and it is important that you do not encourage them to hold out hope that this is the case. Whilst in some ways a delay in obtaining a second opinion can seem to be very unfortunate, many parents will need some time to get used to the idea of what has happened. It is asking too much for someone to go straight from knowing she is pregnant and her baby is alive to knowing that her baby has died. Her mind needs time to adjust to the new reality. As well as this, a couple will not want to be rushed into doing anything that acknowledges that their baby is dead until they are convinced that this is true. They may want to hold on to the belief that the first scan was not true and that the 'mistake' will be revealed by the second scan, so that they have a little more time with the pregnancy, and with their baby, before having to start letting go.

A scan in these circumstances will often show features that demonstrate that the baby has been dead for some time, meaning that the death occurred before the woman's arrival at the hospital, maybe the day before or even earlier. One may see Spalding's sign, in which the skull bones override each other and collapse inwards on the brain, and the spine may be much more curled than usual. Mothers may find it very hard to believe that their baby has died, and even harder to believe that the death may have occurred two or more days ago. They will say that they have been feeling the baby moving, when in fact what they have been feeling is the baby's body moving in the amniotic fluid. It is very important for members of staff to be able to explain this kindly. It is all too easy to talk about the facts of intrauterine death having occurred before the woman arrived at the hospital and make the words sound like a partially veiled or even explicit criticism of her as a woman and a mother. You may think you're saying 'I'm afraid it looks from the scan as if your baby has been dead for a little while' and yet it comes out like 'Surely you must have realised yesterday that your baby wasn't moving. Why did it take you so long to come here?' She may, on some level, have known that there was something wrong and yet could not possibly summon the courage to acknowledge this by presenting at the hospital. You will help her by being kind and sympathetic, not by asking why she did not act sooner or do better. It is also likely that even if she had presented earlier, her baby would still not have survived.

Spontaneous versus induced labour

In a few cases, the labour will start naturally, but in most cases in which an intrauterine death is diagnosed pre-labour, you will need to have a discussion about induction. In our experience, most women will want an induction, saying that they do not want to carry their dead baby any more, but a few will want to wait or will be unable to make up their minds. Unless her clinical condition is giving cause for concern (for example, because of sepsis, severe pre-eclampsia or an abruption), there is no hurry and the woman can be reassured that she will not come to harm by delaying the delivery. She can certainly wait for up to a week without risk of physical harm if this is what she prefers. There is some evidence that waiting over a month would significantly increase her risk of coagulation problems,[1] but it would be unusual for a woman to want to wait this long.

Induction of labour in a case of IUFD

The recommended regimen for induction of labour in a case of IUFD is mifepristone 200 mg orally followed 36–48 hours later by intermittent misoprostol until labour establishes. The initial use of mifepristone in this way reduces the duration of labour.[2] Misoprostol can be given orally or vaginally, but there are fewer side effects with the latter. Some people find the thought of the wait between the mifepristone and the misoprostol intolerable, and it is important that you are able to explain that there are advantages to this regimen in the long run.

Recent guidelines from the National Institute for Health and Clinical Excellence[3] recommend misoprostol 100 mcg 6 hourly before 26 weeks' gestation and 25–50 mcg 4 hourly after 26 weeks. At the time of writing, the tablets available in the UK contain 200 mcg of misoprostol; these can be either cut in half or dissolved in water and divided to achieve the correct dose.

Preparing for the delivery

The woman must be looked after in a room specially designed for the purpose. Whilst you need access to clinical equipment, this can be kept very minimal, and the environment can be made as peaceful and safe as is possible in the circumstances, with comfortable furnishings and soft lighting. There can be a double bed so that the woman's partner can stay with her, and basic niceties such as tea and coffee available.

You must make time to talk to her about what she should expect during the labour, and be prepared to answer all her questions. You need to acknowledge that she may be very frightened at the thought of having to give birth to a dead baby. You should explain what will happen with the misoprostol: how often it is given and how it is administered, and that its effects can be unpredictable, varying from woman to woman. As well as being distressed, she may be very frightened, particularly about how she will cope and about how her baby is likely to look and feel. It is worth mentioning early on that she has a choice about whether to see her baby: she does not have to look straight away or even at all if she does not want to do so. There will be time later to discuss this again, and many women who initially feel that it will be too difficult for them to see their dead babies will gradually become accustomed to the idea and change their minds.

The aim is for you and your colleagues to care for her throughout her labour and delivery and you can tell her that if you have to leave her briefly you will return as soon as you can. This means that you should not be expected to look after any other women, and that when you have your meal break there will be another midwife to look after your patient in your place. This can be challenging for the midwife in charge when it comes to allocating midwives to labouring women on each shift, especially if the unit is busy. We have known of cases in which a midwife was expected to look after a labouring woman with an intrauterine death in one room, and another woman with a live baby down the corridor. This expects far too much of the midwife, who has to be 'schizophrenic' as she goes from one room to the other, and is hugely unfair to both the patients concerned.

Pain relief

Women need to know about the available forms of pain relief before their labour starts, so that they can be reassured that they have a choice, and you need to be able to discuss these. You must try to do so without pushing the woman into agreeing to have one thing or the other. You might choose to have morphine if you were in her shoes, but that does not mean that you should encourage her to have it if she says no. She should also be aware that choosing one type of pain relief does not then exclude the use of others.

A few women may say at first that they do not want any pain relief at all. Others will want pain relief but will want to remain clear-headed throughout the labour and will opt for an epidural, which can be started either before the induction commences or once the labour is established. Blood must be taken for a full blood count to check the platelet level before an epidural is requested to ensure that the woman does not have a coagulopathy, and the anaesthetist must be informed of the result. Some women will want to be drowsy during the labour and will prefer an analgesic that can be a sedative as well. For them, a version of PCA containing morphine with the addition of an anti-emetic may be preferable. Midwives looking after a woman with a PCA must be trained in its use. For example, they need to know how to check for signs of respiratory depression and how to use naloxone to counteract the morphine should this be necessary. Whilst most units will have regular staff training, usually by anaesthetists, in the use of PCA, not all staff may be up to date with their training and it is important that at least one midwife on each shift is appropriately trained.

Management of labour

This is essentially the same as any other labour, except in a few important respects. You should not rupture the membranes artificially, but leave them intact, if possible, to reduce the risk of possible sepsis. If the membranes rupture spontaneously then you can augment labour with oxytocin if necessary. The only monitoring required is of the woman's pulse, blood pressure and temperature. You should gauge the frequency and strength of her contractions by palpation, not with tocography.

Delivery

A dead baby's body is soft and floppy, and it is understandable that many staff will feel anxious about delivering a dead baby because of concern that they will damage the body or, worse, that the body will fall to pieces during the birth. It is unusual for the baby's body to be damaged during the delivery, but she may become bruised or the maceration or skin peeling may become more obvious. You can talk before delivery with the mother about this and find out her ideas about what will happen to the baby during the delivery, so that you can reassure her as much as you can. There is no particular rush to deliver the baby and so no haste is necessary. You can allow the head to descend naturally and wait for the delivery to be completed in its own time. Waiting for the birth to be completed may be very upsetting for the mother, her family and for you, but if the delivery can be achieved without instruments or stitches it will be better for her in the longer term. The natural collapse of the skull bones after the baby's death will mean that moulding of the head is more pronounced and, as a result, the second stage may be quicker than it would have been had her baby been alive.

Sometimes the delivery can be quicker than anyone expects. Estimating the time it will take between the start of the induction and the delivery can often be very inaccurate. We have often heard women describe their babies being born quickly and the midwife being out of the room at the time. We have known of situations in which women have wanted to push, feeling as if they wanted to open their bowels, only to realise that the baby was being born into the toilet.

In some circumstances, the delivery is not straightforward and an obstetrician may need to assist. This is most likely if the baby is very big or if there is a malpresentation. Whoever is carrying out the delivery has to try to deliver the baby carefully without pulling too hard and, if possible, without causing any damage to the baby's body. This is particularly difficult if there is shoulder dystocia; in severe cases, it may be kinder to transfer the mother to the operating theatre so that she can be anaesthetised before her baby is delivered.

If the death occurred a few days before delivery, the liquor may have a very unpleasant smell. You should, of course, try as hard as you can to show that this does not bother you, and reassure the woman that it is normal in the circumstances. Letting her know of this possibility can be part of your pre-labour discussion.

Delivery of a dead baby by Caesarean section (CS)

In a small number of cases, the delivery will be best carried out by CS because of the mother's clinical condition. In other cases, the woman may request a CS because she cannot bear the thought of having to give birth to her dead baby. This requires a sensitive discussion between the mother and a senior obstetrician. The woman has the right to request a CS, but she needs to be made aware of the consequences of this choice, both in terms of her immediate recovery and the implications for future childbirth. If her uterus is scarred, in future she will have to choose between a vaginal birth after caesarean (VBAC), which may or may not be successful, or request another planned CS.

If the woman has had a previous CS and presents with an intrauterine death, a senior consultant should discuss the pros and cons of induction versus delivery by CS. It is still worth giving her mifepristone once the death has been diagnosed, as if she then goes on to choose labour the process will be quicker. The evidence about the risks of induction in the presence of one lower segment scar is based on studies of women having a VBAC with a live baby, and these studies tend to focus on the potential risks to the baby: there are few studies about the risks in similar cases where the baby is dead. One study from Texas[4] of 209 women described a successful VBAC rate of 76% in women with one previous CS and an IUFD, with a 2.4% uterine rupture rate.

If labour is induced, it should be with 25–50 mcg misoprostol; however, even with these small doses, 1% of women are likely to have problems with their uterine scar[5] and should be warned of this and told what to expect should this happen. The risks of complications when inducing labour in women who have had two lower segment sections is slightly greater than after one, with 3.2% of women having major problems including scar rupture.[6]

Women with vertical uterine incisions, from a classical CS or an open myomectomy, have an unpredictable risk of scar rupture if labour is induced, and should be delivered by CS.

THE PLACENTA

Histological examination of the placenta, whether it is delivered normally or has to be removed manually, can be extremely helpful in determining the reason for the baby's death. This can be done whether or not the parents request a PM examination of the baby. Tests on the placenta are discussed in more detail in Chapter 10, 'Tests, post-mortems and paperwork'.

AFTER THE DELIVERY

The usual post-delivery observations need to be done, in the same way as if the woman had delivered a live baby. It is a challenge to check for a contracted uterus and normal lochia in these circumstances because you are trying to be practical in the midst of so much emotion, but the timely performance of these checks is a vital part of making sure the woman recovers safely. The checks have to be carried out in the context of letting the couple be with their baby and if you are gentle and careful they may hardly notice what you are doing.

All women who have delivered a dead baby must be given cabergoline 1 mg within 24 hours (preferably sooner) of the delivery, to inhibit lactation and prevent the pain and distress of breasts filling with milk. Cabergoline works well as long as the breasts are not stimulated, and has very few side effects compared with its predecessor bromocriptine.

Various people need to be told about the loss. These include the woman's GP, the antenatal clinic and scan department (so that they stop sending her appointments) and the community midwives, so that they are aware of the situation when they go to visit the woman after she has been discharged from hospital. The task of telling these people may fall to the midwife who is looking after the woman or the labour ward clerk, but there must be clarity about who is doing it so that it does not get overlooked.

MAKING THIS PROCESS MORE BEARABLE FOR YOURSELF

There are simple things that you can do to help deal with this process. As we have already said, if you are the midwife assigned to care for a woman giving birth to a dead baby, you should only be looking after this woman and no one else. The senior midwife in charge of the labour ward must make sure that you have the breaks you are entitled to and that another midwife is available to care for the woman in your absence. You should make the most of your break by trying to eat well and getting outside in the fresh air if this is possible.

You need to learn the art of compartmentalisation within your mind, so that you can function successfully at work without becoming overwhelmed by emotion and, equally, carry on a normal life outside work without dwelling too much on the sadness you have had to endure that day. It is an art that comes more readily to some than to others, but which usually becomes easier with time and practice. Being able to compartmentalise in this way does not make you an unfeeling individual; it is a skill that equips you to deal with others' tragedies and clinical emergencies professionally and correctly.

SUMMARY

We have been told over and over again about how much of a difference midwives and doctors make when they are kind and consistent during the delivery of a dead baby. Women often talk about their caregivers in this situation in remarkably warm and generous terms. Women remember and appreciate when they have been looked after kindly: they will say 'it was a terrible time, but I felt really cared for'. This is in contrast to those who describe the same events but with different staff by saying 'they just made a terrible time worse'. It is very important to realise that you can make a huge difference to the woman and her family during this ordeal, and there is a great satisfaction to be gained by managing this situation well.

It is also important to know that you are not jinxed, or some kind of bad fairy, if you are often asked to look after bereaved women. You are probably being asked because you are good at it. We have known women who came back to the same unit where they lost a baby, having chosen the same midwife who delivered the dead baby to deliver their next (live) child, so closing a loop in a very special way for all concerned.

REFERENCES

1. Parasnis H, Raje B, Hinduja IN. Relevance of plasma fibrinogen estimation in obstetric complications. *J Postgrad Med.* 1992; **38**(4): 183–5.
2. Wagaarachchi PT, Ashok PW, Narvekar N *et al.* Medical management of late intrauterine death using a combination of mifepristone and misoprostol. *BJOG.* 2002; **109**(4): 443–7.
3. National Institute for Health and Clinical Excellence (NIHCE). *Induction of Labour: NICE guideline 70.* London: NIHCE; 2008. www.nice.org.uk/nicemedia/pdf/CG070NICEGuideline.pdf
4. Ramirez MM, Gilbert S, Landon MB *et al.* Mode of delivery in women with antepartum fetal death and prior cesarean delivery. *Am J Perinatol.* 2010; **27**(10): 825–30.
5. Landon MB, Hauth JC, Leveno KJ *et al.* Maternal and perinatal outcomes associated with a trial of labor after prior cesarean delivery. *N Engl J Med.* 2004; **351**(25): 2581–9.
6. Macones GA, Cahill A, Pare E *et al.* Obstetric outcomes in women with two prior cesarean deliveries: is vaginal birth after cesarean delivery a viable option? *Am J Obstet Gynecol.* 2005; **192**(4): 1223–8, discussion 1228–9.

CHAPTER 8

When something goes wrong in labour

INTRODUCTION

This chapter focuses on the particularly difficult issue of unexpected intrapartum death. We discuss how staff wonder, as mothers do, 'Could I have done something differently?' It is difficult to imagine a more appalling experience for a woman than going to a maternity unit in labour, happily expecting the imminent arrival of her baby, only to have to leave later without her baby because he has suddenly and unexpectedly died. We discuss various aspects of this terrible event, from the initial diagnosis, through the management of the birth and then on to the aftermath.

Sudden intrapartum death will usually be related to either a fetal bradycardia or a placental abruption. In both cases, there may be absolutely no warning. One minute the labour is progressing as expected and the next minute the emergency buzzer has been pressed and there is serious concern or even panic. Alternatively, there may have been warning signs: the cardiotocograph (CTG) recording may have been abnormal for some time before the bradycardia, or the woman may have been complaining of pain between her contractions before collapsing with an abruption. Any senior member of staff talking to patients after an intrapartum death must look carefully at the events leading up to the death to try to make sense of what has happened. In particular, they must be prepared for patients to say, 'we knew that something was wrong' or, worse, 'we tried to tell the staff that something was wrong, but they said that everything was okay'. If this is the case, the patient's and her partner's accounts must be explored and noted.

CTG INTERPRETATION

CTG interpretation is a basic skill required of every midwife and doctor involved in intrapartum care. Most trusts have some form of mandatory training programme in CTG interpretation, which will either be an in-house or external web-based scheme. It is important, from the perspective of clinical governance and the Clinical Negligence Scheme for Trusts, to be able to demonstrate that maternity unit staff have taken part in this training. There is, however, a big difference between answering questions in a seminar room or on a website about how to describe a particular section of CTG, and actually looking at a CTG in a labour that you have been monitoring for several hours and noticing the subtle changes that might herald a pathological trace. It might be that the previously normal baseline variability became reduced by more than could be explained by fetal sleep, or the baseline rate very gradually increased over the course of 2 hours. A contraction pattern that gradually changes from a normal rate of three or four times every 10 minutes to small contractions every minute might be displaying the signs of abruption before the patient does. Noticing these changes takes training, concentration and an eye for detail, and it is a particular challenge when you are being asked to do too many things at once. If, after changes such as this, there is a sudden bradycardia that does not recover, the CTG will be carefully scrutinised by senior members of staff after the event and you will be asked 'Didn't you notice these changes?' It is always easy to be wise with hindsight. Nonetheless, fetal monitoring should mean just that: we are monitoring the fetus and we are especially looking out for signs that things are not as they were before.

It is so important to check the mother's pulse at the start of a CTG, to differentiate it from her baby's. We have seen instances in which women have been told that their baby must have died before their labour began, but the mothers are convinced that this could not be the case because 'staff were monitoring the baby's heartbeat during labour'. If the mother is tachycardic, perhaps because of anxiety or pain, with a pulse rate of, say, between 110 and 120 beats per minute, it is possible to obtain a perfectly normal looking CTG that actually represents the mother's heartbeat pattern and not that of her baby. We know this because when a stillborn baby is macerated, she must have been dead *in utero* for at least 24 hours, so the 'fetal' heartbeat was in fact the mother's. This is fairly simple for staff to understand in hindsight but is very difficult for patients to accept, as they will have been convinced that it was their baby's heartbeat they were hearing because this is what they were told. They will have trusted the staff to monitor it correctly. Acknowledging the mistake is very important for all concerned, but the conversation required to explain this to bereaved parents is a challenging one.

For some women, especially obese women, obtaining an accurate CTG can be very difficult because there will be loss of contact between the Doppler fetal monitor part of the CTG apparatus and the fetal heart. It is wise for a midwife or obstetrician to tell obese women during the antenatal period that they may warrant a fetal scalp electrode (FSE) during labour if continuous monitoring of the fetal heart rate is required. We know of a case in which there was intermittent loss of contact using an external monitor during an obese woman's labour over the course of several hours. By the time the staff realised that there had been so much loss of contact, it was too late to save the baby. A subsequent detailed assessment of the CTG during the labour showed that, whilst the fetal heart had been present in the early stages, there were many sections later when there was loss of contact and it was during one of these periods that her baby died.

There may also be problems with loss of contact if the woman is moving about a great deal. If the mother needs continuous monitoring and she is moving, an effective external CTG trace will be impossible to achieve. It will be better to attach an FSE, especially if the situation has become more complicated – for example, because of meconium in the liquor.

Most importantly, if a patient requires continuous monitoring, then her midwife needs to look at the CTG in real time, ideally in the same room as the labouring woman. Sometimes staffing levels on the labour ward make this a challenge, but there is no point in 'monitoring' if no one is watching.

CSS FOR CTG ABNORMALITIES AND OTHER EMERGENCIES

There is a difference between recognising that a previously normal fetal heartbeat pattern has changed suddenly into a non-recovering bradycardia, and a prolonged abnormal CTG that becomes terminal and fades away to nothing whilst no one notices. In the first scenario, there is a potential chance to save the baby with a Category 1 CS. The category system is a way of communicating the urgency of the case to other staff. Category 1 means that the baby should be born within 30 minutes of the decision to deliver being made; Category 2 means deliver within 60 minutes of the decision; Category 3 means aim to deliver within 75 minutes. The so-called 3-minute rule of managing a sudden bradycardia (3 minutes to diagnose the bradycardia, 3 more minutes to recognise it and start doing something about it, 3 minutes to get the patient to theatre and ready for a GA and 3 minutes to deliver the baby) requires continuous electronic fetal monitoring with one-to-one care by someone who can interpret the CTG and press the emergency buzzer in a timely fashion.

In the second scenario, for example, when no one has been looking at the monitor for a while and it is clear that the fetal heart stopped beating over 15 minutes or more ago, it is unlikely that immediate delivery will save the baby, although many would still try. We have known of women who have been subjected to a Category 1 CS in this sort of case: some of the patients said that they realised at the time that there was no point in doing this but felt that the staff did not want to believe it. Others were grateful that the staff 'tried their best' and did not seem to mind that they had major surgery for what turned out to be a lost cause.

Are there situations when we should agree to a CS even though we think that the case for the baby is hopeless? Equally, should we encourage a vaginal delivery even if there is a small chance that the baby would fare better if delivered by CS? Generally speaking, the mother will want to do what she perceives as being right for her baby, whereas staff tend to have a wider view and would always put the mother first. This dilemma can arise with a very preterm breech baby. Suppose the mother is in labour at 25 weeks' gestation with ruptured membranes and a breech presentation. There is evidence that preterm breech babies do better if delivered by CS, but the prognosis for a baby born at 25 weeks' gestation, who may already be infected, is very poor. The baby may die during labour or soon afterwards, and if he survives he may well be severely damaged. The mother may ask for a CS and after discussion with her the most senior member of staff has either to agree or refuse, gently, and be prepared to defend the decision later. If, as the senior doctor present, you agree, you must do your very best to make the risks from the surgery and anaesthetic clear to the mother as well as the implications for future deliveries and the potential problems for the newborn baby. If you genuinely feel that there is no chance that the baby will survive, you must explain carefully why you believe this to be the case and document your points in the patient's notes. Efforts should be made to communicate as well as possible in this difficult situation, and the conversations, because there will be more than one of them, must include a neonatologist as well as an obstetrician and a midwife.

CHOICE OF ANAESTHESIA

A Category 1 CS does not always mean a GA. To some extent, it depends on your anaesthetic colleague, since with a Category 1 CS you probably do not have time to call in anyone else. If the obstetric anaesthetist on call with you is reliably quick, she or he will have sited a spinal in the time it takes you to scrub and gown up for the operation. That said, a regional technique may not always be suitable – say, if the patient is bleeding heavily and her blood pressure is falling, or if the patient is too terrified to keep still. GA sections are a challenge for our anaesthetic colleagues, and junior anaesthetists should summon support from a consultant if called upon to do an emergency GA section. This is especially true if the mother's condition is serious – for example, if there has been a uterine rupture or severe post-partum haemorrhage.

If the woman has to have a GA and there is uncertainty about the baby's chance of survival, the couple are very rapidly faced with a terrible challenge. Neither will witness the baby's birth, since the mother will be unconscious and the father will not be in the operating theatre with her. It may well be the case that the father will see the baby alive, but the mother may not do so if her baby dies before she wakes up from the anaesthetic. She will have to hear her partner's view of what happened and have to rely upon his interpretation of the events. This may chime with the interpretation given by the staff, but may not, and you should be prepared for confusion at best and conflict at worst.

If you know that the baby is already dead, there is of course more time for discussion. In these circumstances, it may be that it is kinder for all concerned if the woman is asleep, but she should still be offered the choice if at all possible.

KEEPING PATIENTS INFORMED

For some staff, it is perhaps a natural reaction to want to stay away from a patient who is in difficulty. A part of us would rather not be involved and in fact would rather be anywhere but in the same room as her. The whole idea is worrying and possibly frightening. When confronted by a patient who has, for example, just given birth to a baby who has been born alive but who has been whisked away to the neonatal unit with little hope of a good prognosis, we can easily feel a variety of emotions, all of which conspire to make us feel useless. We do not know what to say; we are afraid of saying the wrong thing; we are afraid of saying anything at all in case we make matters worse; we are afraid we will be to blame; we are afraid we may inadvertently blame others; we would rather not be associated with this awful situation. But no matter how difficult it is, we need to overcome our fears.

Imagine how much worse it is for the woman, who is desperate to know what has happened to her baby and cannot understand why no one is talking to her. We have known of a woman who was left alone in the recovery room for more than 2 hours after a difficult instrumental delivery, not knowing what was going on or where her partner was. Her baby was in the neonatal unit, the labour ward was busy and the midwife concerned with her case had been told to do her paperwork and had chosen, perhaps out of anxiety, to do this in another room. It is easy to see how the woman gets lost in this maelstrom, but it is vitally important to keep her informed. She needs to know where her baby is, what has happened so far and what to expect next, and when she will be able to see her baby for herself. If you do not know the answers to all these questions, you should at least be able to say something like 'the baby doctors are looking after your baby, and I will go and talk to them and come back as soon as I can to tell you what is happening' *and then actually do this.*

It is so important for the mother to see her baby, even if only fleetingly, before he is taken in the incubator to the neonatal unit, as this may be the only chance she has of doing so whilst he is still alive. We know of women who never saw their babies alive because the neonatal team, understandably, were anxious to get the baby to the neonatal unit as soon as possible and pushed the transport incubator quickly out of the operating theatre without stopping to show the mother. This action was obviously full of good intention but served to haunt the women after their babies had died. They have told us that they feel that in some way they may have been able to help their babies if only they had had a chance to see them. One woman told us 'if only I could have seen him, perhaps I could have passed on some of my strength to him to help him, but I never had the chance'.

The pressures on neonatal units mean that babies, especially very sick ones, may be transferred to another hospital, perhaps a long way from the mother. Whilst efforts are made to keep the two together, this may be difficult if the mother is also very unwell and too unstable to be moved straight away. This can make life extremely difficult for the baby's father and other relatives, and staff must bear the practical considerations in mind as well as the clinical and emotional ones.

KEEPING RELATIVES INFORMED

As far as possible, you must keep a patient's relatives informed about what is going on if events become complicated or risky, especially if the patient has to go to theatre without a relative accompanying her, for example, if she is under a GA. It may not be appropriate for a senior clinician to talk to relatives as the case progresses, since he or she will be busy dealing with the actual case, perhaps trying to control a haemorrhage or helping with attempts to resuscitate the baby. If this is the case, then someone, perhaps a manager who is not clinically involved, should talk to the relatives to keep them up to date with what is happening without straying into complex clinical territory or betraying any confidences. Relatives should be given a realistic time frame: for example, a woman's parents might be told 'your daughter will be in the operating theatre for at least an hour, and will be kept in the recovery room until she is awake. You will be able to see her then but that may be 2 hours from now.' They should be told enough to take the situation seriously but not too much before the reality of the case is clear. There are some stock phrases that are often used, for example, 'the doctors are doing everything they can', which may well be true, but which sound like lines from a bad television hospital drama, and are probably best avoided.

As soon as it is feasible, the most senior clinician present should talk to the family members and explain simply and clearly what has happened and what to expect. This should be in a quiet place out of earshot from other patients and their relatives. Whoever talks to the relatives should have someone else present who can help with practical things like making tea, passing on contact telephone numbers, or helping with directions, say, to the recovery room. If you have been clinically involved and then go to talk to relatives, spare a moment first to think about how you appear as well as about what you will say. I (Ruth) remember going to talk to a woman's husband after I had dealt successfully with her severe post-partum haemorrhage. The first thing he noticed was the blood on my theatre clogs and he told me later that he had immediately concluded from this that his wife had bled to death.

If a baby has unexpectedly died, and his mother does not yet know because she is still under anaesthetic, it is correct to tell the baby's father about what has happened. However, it is not fair to tell other members of her family about the death until you have been able to talk to her, unless the mother's clinical situation is so precarious that you have no choice.

PRACTICAL TASKS AFTER AN INTRAPARTUM DEATH

Good documentation is a basic requirement of good clinical care. With documentation, the patient's story, from the staff's point of view at least, can be told and our care can be judged. If a case has been difficult or complex and when the outcome is a perinatal death, it is particularly important that the clinical notes are clear, unambiguous and complete. Notes should, in an ideal world, be written contemporaneously, but, as one of our midwifery colleagues says, 'you can't deliver a baby and write your notes at the same time'. Notes written in retrospect must be clearly stated as such and should be written as soon after the events as possible. It is not appropriate to go home after dealing with a case without completing your notes, intending to write them the next day. Your colleagues will need to know what has happened and will need to be able to read your notes so that they can carry on caring for the patient safely. If you have to stay beyond the end of your shift to write your notes, your manager should ensure that you have the time back at a later date.

An intrapartum death is a serious clinical incident and one of the team must report it. It does not matter if more than one person reports it as long as someone does, using a special form that, depending on your trust, will be either paper or electronic.

Dealing with intrapartum death is another example of when you need a way of compartmentalising your brain. In this situation, you need to be practical and dextrous when delivering the baby; kind, sympathetic and patient when talking with the bereaved parents and other family members; organised and efficient when completing the paperwork and other administrative duties that attend perinatal death; clear-headed and perhaps slightly suspicious when considering the risk management aspects of the case. By this we mean that difficult cases can make some members of staff feel very threatened and they may then seek to try to hide or diminish their involvement by altering notes or removing the printouts from the CTG machine if they feel that these might incriminate them in some way. There have been too many instances of notes being altered and CTG traces going missing after a loss for this not to be true. It is an understandable, though misguided, panicky reaction to a terrible event and will always be found out.

If you are involved in an intrapartum death, a serious incident will be declared and you will be required by your trust to write a statement about your involvement. All those involved will be asked to do so. It is important, therefore, that the notes (including the CTGs) are copied for distribution to the relevant staff members. Usually one of the administrative staff will be asked to do this, but it is good practice to make a copy of the CTG – if there is one – yourself as soon as possible in case this is lost from the main notes. The copy can be used for teaching purposes later and can be helpful if the original version 'goes missing'.

You should write your statement as soon as possible after the event, perhaps even before you have been asked to do so. In this way, you can put in all the necessary details whilst they are still fresh and clear in your mind. You must write a purely factual account of your own involvement; you should not pass any judgement on the actions of others or give opinions about what you think has happened. It is sensible to include any contextual detail that is relevant to your involvement in the case. For example, you should state if the activity on the labour ward was such that you were expected to look after two different women and could not leave one to help the other straight away. Another example would be if you were a doctor dealing with a patient with an ectopic pregnancy whilst also being on call for the labour ward.

Serious incident reports allow hospitals to review their practices and to learn from difficult cases. They are also very important to patients, a fact that needs to be understood by those who compile the reports. There is always a deadline for the production of these reports and any delay in their completion and, therefore, in the patient's receipt of their copy of the report, will add insult to the patient's injury and may increase their suspicion that there has been some sort of cover-up.

SENIOR SUPPORT

You need the support of senior colleagues when dealing with a rare and serious situation like an intrapartum death. Hopefully, a senior colleague will either be dealing with the case alongside you or will be immediately contactable and available. If this is not the case then you have the right to ask for senior help, both at the time and afterwards. There will be aspects of the care that you may wish to carry out yourself, especially if you have been looking after the woman from the time of her admission and have got to know her; alternatively, there may be things that you feel should be done by someone more senior, for example, telling a woman's partner that their baby has unexpectedly been born dead. Carrying out these painful duties does not become easier as you become more senior, because it is always painful, but there is at least the benefit of familiarity and experience. It is helpful for senior staff to take a junior colleague with them in situations like this, as a way of demonstrating how to talk and behave and as a way of perhaps defusing some of the ideas the junior colleague might have about how awful it will be.

Senior medical staff rarely have support, other than from their senior medical colleagues, and then usually only if it is explicitly requested. Recently appointed consultant staff will be able to rely upon more senior colleagues, and midwives have the help of a supervisor to whom they can turn.

BEING OPEN AND HONEST

It hopefully goes without saying that you should be honest with patients when something has gone wrong. It is, however, extremely difficult and many patients talk about staff seeming evasive, embarrassed or even obstructive after a disaster when asked for explanations. Honesty is crucial; patients will know straight away if you are not telling the truth or if you are hiding something. If you feel unable to be honest and truthful with patients, especially if they are asking questions about an unexpected tragedy, you must ask for senior help.

Openness and honesty are important both at the time of the death and during any meetings afterwards. Even though the death is being investigated as a serious incident, this is not a reason for withholding information about the death from the parents. The fact that an investigation is underway does not prevent senior clinicians from communicating kindly with the parents about what happened, how they are feeling and what advice they can be offered. You should see two parallel lines of communication in these cases: one in which the parents are counselled and offered both clinical explanation and sympathetic help, and another in which the case is investigated so that, if necessary, the trust can learn lessons from the case. Two senior clinicians will be involved, one to sympathise with the parents and explain what is happening and the other to lead the investigation.

Senior staff may find that colleagues in the patient advice and liaison service or complaints department have useful insights in these situations, as they will be used to hearing patients talk about what went wrong. Colleagues from the legal department will have at least one eye on any possible future litigation in such cases but will still recognise the importance of being completely frank with bereaved patients and their relatives.

The National Patient Safety Agency[1] has for some years encouraged the practice of 'being open' and has useful information to support staff in this task.

BLAME

When something unexpectedly bad happens in pregnancy there will be those who blame themselves. Patients do this a lot, as we have said before: 'I shouldn't have lifted that heavy box/had that glass of wine/worked such long shifts.' Members of staff often do this too, blaming themselves when there is nothing they could have done to change the situation. They will feel convinced that they missed something, or that they did not try hard enough, or that they did not ask for help soon enough, even though none of this may be true.

Sometimes the patient is blamed (not to her face, of course) for not having done something or not having noticed sooner that something was wrong. An example of this would be the woman who arrives on the labour ward saying that she has not felt her baby move for the past 2 days. The staff know that she should have presented sooner and it requires a lot of tact to be able to ask gentle questions about what the woman was thinking without making an already horrible situation worse.

Others will blame other people, perhaps not individuals explicitly, but 'the rota', 'the cuts', 'the managers'. They may have a point, but those who blame others in this way may be doing their best, consciously or subconsciously, to deflect blame away from themselves: 'How could I be expected to have noticed that pre-terminal CTG if I was being asked to look after three women at once?' This begs a question about why staffing levels were that risky and whether enough had been done to alert senior managers to the potential problems of an inadequate staffing roster.

It may be that a member of staff will be blamed for not escalating a problem or not doing so quickly enough. For example, well-meaning middle-grade doctors may try to handle a serious situation themselves without summoning senior help, as they believe that they can manage the case and do not want to 'bother' the consultant. The consultant, of course, needs to be bothered if the situation warrants it, and other junior medical staff and midwives should feel able to call the consultant themselves if the registrar has not yet done so. It is far better that a consultant is called in a timely fashion than summoned once the case has become disastrous.

You might be unfairly blamed by the patient or by other members of staff for having neglected to do something or failing to notice something. Alternatively, it may be that, to some extent at least, you *are* to blame when something goes wrong. If this is the case, you should talk about it with a senior colleague. It may be that what you did or did not do did not actually change the outcome of the case, and talking to someone more experienced may help you to realise this.

A senior member of staff will feel responsible when something goes wrong, even if she or he was not personally to blame for what happened. The fact that you are the most senior person on call means that you will feel that you *should* have been told, you *should* have known what to do and you *should* have been able to do something. Most senior members of staff are good at telling their colleagues that something 'was not their fault', but we are not very good at saying this to ourselves. Your senior position means that you accept responsibility when things go wrong, even if there was nothing that you could have done to have made a difference. Accepting responsibility is not the same thing as being to blame.

DEBRIEFING

Given all the above, after a particularly difficult case, it is helpful for all those who were personally involved to get together to talk about what happened. Ideally, this should be arranged soon after the event, certainly within a couple of days, and should, if possible, be facilitated by someone who was not involved and who can be independent and objective. If you are involved in organising a debriefing meeting, you should try hard to include everybody, remembering that this may mean contacting people outside of your immediate work environment. For example, if a woman was brought into hospital with an abruption after which her baby died, you may wish to include the paramedics in the ambulance, the theatre team and the neonatal staff as well as the midwives and obstetricians who were on duty at the time. You may find that people are able to learn from each other during the meeting and empathise better with their colleagues afterwards, having shared such a powerful and difficult experience. Just as patients need to be listened to, so staff need to be able to explore both their actions and their feelings in a non-judgemental setting.

TALKING TO YOUR DEFENCE ORGANISATION

If you are personally involved in the care of a patient in which there has been a poor outcome, especially if the mother or her baby has been seriously harmed or has died, regardless of whether mistakes have been made, it would be wise to inform your defence organisation. This will be the Medical Defence Union (MDU)[2] or the Medical Protection Society (MPS)[3] for doctors and the Nursing and Midwifery Council (NMC)[4] for nurses and midwives. It will do no harm to inform them and they will be a very valuable source of support and practical advice at a difficult time. If the case proceeds, perhaps with a complaint and a claim, then you already have a professional independent source of support. It may also be that you feel able to talk more easily about your concerns to your advisor at the MDU, MPS or the NMC than you could to a close friend or a colleague.

ACCEPTANCE

If you have been involved in an intrapartum death, it is initially very difficult to get the details out of your mind and you may find it hard to detach yourself from the case. You may feel as though you are a jinx and that your actions or even just your presence made something terrible happen. Most departments have had a member of staff who, through no fault of their own, is unfortunate enough to be involved in a string of perinatal loss cases. If you are in this position, you may feel as if you are the cause of the problem and that you have some responsibility for what has happened. If these thoughts were to persist, you would not be able to go back on duty. You have to find some way of putting those thoughts in a place in your mind that allows you to process them whilst at the same time carrying on with your work. Usually this will be by talking with a colleague, preferably one with enough experience to be able to help you put your feelings into some kind of perspective. If talking to your colleagues, family or friends does not help, then your trust should provide you with access to services such as counselling through which you will be able to reflect in a safe, non-judgemental environment.

SUMMARY

Caring for women when something goes wrong in labour is a hard task and a huge responsibility. If some aspects of your care require improvement or further training, then you must accept this with patience and humility. If you still feel to blame, even if whatever happened was not really your fault, you may find that similar cases bring feelings of heightened awareness and anxiety. If you can learn to harness that awareness then you will be mentally prepared to deal with these cases as well as you possibly can. By doing this, you will learn from past experiences rather than being rendered helpless by them.

REFERENCES

1. www.nrls.npsa.nhs.uk
2. www.the-mdu.com
3. www.medicalprotection.org
4. www.nmc-uk.org

CHAPTER 9

What to do with the baby

INTRODUCTION

This chapter deals with helping parents to see and hold their dead baby, and gives some suggestions about how you can create an environment in which memories can be built and parents can be helped to grieve.

SEEING AND HOLDING THE BABY

It has become standard practice to show parents their dead baby and to encourage them to hold their baby in a natural way. This would have been unthinkable two generations ago. It used to be the case that dead babies were taken away from their mothers as soon as they were delivered, never to be seen again, and the bereaved woman was left imagining how her baby would have looked. We know that the images a person can create in their mind are usually far more horrific than the reality, but for many women who lost babies in the mid-twentieth century, it was those images that remained to haunt them.

When a woman knows that she is going to give birth to her baby who has died, you can have a conversation beforehand about how she feels about seeing her baby. Some will say straight away that they do not want to do so, and others will know that they want to or will have an open mind. Whilst seeing the baby has become commonplace, it is important not to be coercive about this. If a woman has told you that she does not want to see her baby, it may be best to put that conversation to one side for the time being and perhaps ask gently, once the baby has been delivered, whether she has changed her mind. There will be time throughout her stay in hospital, and once she has gone home, for her to change her mind.

It is unreasonable to expect a woman or a couple to deal with seeing their baby on their own without help, unless this is what they have told you they want. For most people, the process of seeing their dead baby for the first time will be made much easier if you are able to help them. You might want to move the baby to another room so that you can look at the baby yourself first, away from the couple, to check for any obvious external abnormalities, so you are not taken by surprise when you are showing the baby to the parents. You can tell the parents before the birth that you might do this and find out whether they are agreeable.

It is probably best to start with the baby wrapped in a little towel or blanket, with just her face showing, so that they can hold her in a natural way then, when they are ready, unwrapping the blanket and showing their baby to them. Little hands and feet can be gradually uncovered and, when the parents are ready, they can see the rest of their baby if they wish. You do not need to say very much and, if you do say anything, choose your words with care. When I (Ruth) was a registrar, I remember being with a father when he looked at his stillborn baby daughter. As he cradled her in his arms, I quietly said to him 'she looks perfect' and he looked up and corrected me, saying 'she *is* perfect'.

You may wish to wash the baby gently, either before showing her to the parents or after they have seen her for the first time. Parents may want to help you do this or do it themselves. Washing the baby can make a difference to how parents relate to the baby and to how they feel when they look at photographs later. Babies will often have hair that looks unnaturally dark because of blood or amniotic fluid, but which will show its real colour when washed.

Some parents will be extremely private in their dealings with their baby, but others will involve close family members including, often, the baby's grandparents and siblings. The inclusion of children in this process is again something that was discouraged in past years but which is now seen as a normal and healthy family response. Children will have their own ideas about how their dead baby brother or sister will look and it can help them in the future if they have seen the reality rather than a conjured image.

If the baby's grandparents ask to see the baby, you should check first that the parents are in agreement. Assuming that they agree, they may all want to see the baby together or you may find it easier for everyone if the grandparents see the baby in another room, away from the parents. If this is the case, then you should go with them, so that you can gently tell them what to expect and help them to look at and handle their grandchild, if this is what they want to do. This is a very moving and emotional time in the life of the family and you are privileged to be able to share in it, even though the circumstances can be so upsetting for all concerned.

We recently looked after a couple whose twins died during the second trimester and all the family, including grandparents and aunts of the babies, came to see them. Both babies were lying together in a Moses basket and we were able to show them to their relatives who were together in a tearful but dignified family group. The tone struck by the older family members was particularly moving, especially considering that seeing dead babies in this way was something that was frowned upon when they were younger.

DOCUMENTING HOW THE BABY LOOKS

It is important that one of the doctors on duty at the time the baby is delivered looks carefully at the baby and documents the external appearance in the mother's notes. This must include turning the baby over to look at his back in case he has spina bifida. A good description of the baby's external appearance, written in the mother's notes at the time, is invaluable for anyone seeing the parents for follow-up, especially if the couple decide not to have a PM examination carried out on their baby. A baby that looks normal almost always *is* normal. Alternatively, distinctive external abnormalities may suggest a congenital syndrome that might explain the death.

In cases of preterm membrane rupture, when the baby has been in the uterus with very little or no liquor for some time, the baby's head will appear flattened and the facial features distorted as a result. It would be easy to think that the baby had some form of abnormality, but the appearance will just be the result of pressure on the face from the uterine wall.

A baby that has been dead *in utero* for more than 24 hours will start to become macerated; that is, the skin will start to peel in various places. The extent of the maceration is roughly proportional to the length of time that has passed since the baby died. When it is known that the death occurred more than one day ago, you should prepare the parents for this, as maceration will be likely and obvious. It is important for parents to know that this is a natural phenomenon and not the result of the baby's body being roughly handled during the delivery or afterwards. You should use the term 'skin peeling' rather than 'maceration', a word that can have more sinister connotations.

SEX AND IDENTITY

Knowing whether their baby is a boy or a girl helps parents see their baby in a particular light, with a particular identity. Knowing the sex allows parents to give their baby a name, which in itself acknowledges the baby as a person. When talking about their baby it allows them to say 'he' or 'she' rather than 'it'. They can think about how he or she would have looked and behaved. They can say things like 'she used to lie right on my bladder'; 'he had a really strong kick'; 'she looked just like her sister'.

During early fetal development, it is not possible to determine a baby's sex with the naked eye. Later, during the second trimester, there are a few weeks when female genitalia look masculine. This is because of the relative enlargement of the clitoris and clitoral hood, making it look like a little penis. Therefore, it is often difficult to be sure whether a baby is male or female, especially between 16 and 20 weeks' gestation. A glance at the baby's genital area when the legs are together will show a swelling that looks like a penis when it is in fact a clitoris. To be certain of a baby's sex at this stage you need to look carefully, in a good light, with the baby's legs apart, to see whether there is an open vulva rather than a closed scrotal sac. A few babies will genuinely have ambiguous genitalia and their sex may only be established for certain by karyotyping.

Without this careful examination, blunders can occur. Imagine the scenario of a couple losing a baby at 19 weeks' gestation and being told by the staff that their baby was a little boy. Having been told that their baby was male, they will have given him a name, dressed him in blue clothes and perhaps put a little blue teddy in the Moses basket, thinking of him in a masculine way. His parents might speculate about whether he would have been mischievous like his brother or about which football team he would have supported. All of these thoughts and ideas will have helped the parents to see their baby in a way that makes sense to them, helping them to create a character for him that enables them to grieve a genuine little person. Imagine, then, that they discover, perhaps because of a sharp-eyed mortician or later as a result of PM findings, that their baby was actually a little girl. The character that they have created so lovingly for their little boy has to be taken down and reconstructed for this new, female, person. Everything has to be re-thought, re-characterised, re-mourned.

The implications of misdiagnosing sex are profound for the parents. To be told that they have lost a baby boy only later to discover that they have actually lost a girl (it is, in our experience, always this way round, because of the anatomical issues we have just described) can add another insult to the injury of the loss. It means that they have to start all over again when thinking about their baby, constructing an identity for her and imagining who she would have been. They will have to tell their family and friends that the little boy they have all been grieving was in fact a little girl and the process has to stop and restart for everyone.

If you are in any doubt at all about a baby's sex, it is much better to say something like 'I'm afraid I'm not sure if your baby is a boy or a girl. It is often very difficult to be certain at this stage and I would not want to tell you the wrong sex.' This is perfectly true and you would in no way be avoiding your responsibility. You can make it clear to the parents that if you are not certain of the baby's sex, you will get someone more senior who may be able to tell by examining the baby carefully. If, in turn, the senior colleague is not sure, the sex can be established, with the parents' permission, by taking a small skin sample and testing the baby's chromosomes.

NAMING THE BABY

It is not necessary for parents to give their baby a name, and the giving of a name is not a legal requirement or a prerequisite for burial or cremation, but many will wish to do so. Clearly, the baby's sex is an important consideration when choosing a name, and if the sex is not obvious on examination then a name may have to wait until after a chromosome test or a PM. Some parents may choose a name that would be suitable for either sex or may pick a name such as the day of the week or the season when their baby was born.

If parents have told you their baby's name, it is considerate to use it when referring to their baby and to write her name in the notes and on her cot card and wristbands. It is a kind and polite way of acknowledging that she is a person in the eyes of her parents and wider family.

Some parents find choosing a name for the baby difficult. They may have had names in mind already, but when the baby dies they may find they do not want to use the name they had planned because they had always thought they would use that name for a live baby.

DRESSING THE BABY

Some parents will want to dress their baby with clothes that they have brought with them. Parents often worry that they may damage their baby's body because it feels so fragile, and it is important to handle the baby's body as gently as possible, especially if it is very macerated. They may want to put clothes on their baby themselves but they may ask for your help. Try to be as natural as possible if this is the case, even though the circumstances are so difficult. Loose clothes are the easiest to handle, so that skin is not sloughed off when sleeves are pulled up, for example. A dead baby's head is often misshapen, with the loose skull bones feeling as if they might break, and a little hat or bonnet is very useful for hiding this and framing the face in a suitable way. Any obvious abnormality can be disguised or hidden with clothes or a nicely wrapped shawl so that the baby appears peaceful and looks suitable for photographs and viewing by other family members.

Very tiny babies are too small to wear even newborn baby clothes. Many hospitals have a supply of tiny clothes bought or knitted by volunteers or members of the hospital's league of friends. In our unit, we have some tiny tabards made by the partner of one of our colleagues, which are easy to put on to very small babies.

MEMENTOES AND PHOTOGRAPHS

When a baby dies, the parents will often be very anxious to keep any tangible evidence of their baby's existence. They may have already started to do this long before they imagined the baby might die, with an album of photographs from antenatal ultrasound scans. If they have not got copies of scan photographs, it may be possible to access them on the hospital's radiology computer system where the images are likely to have been stored. We have known many couples who have been surprised and pleased to know that they could have photos of their baby's scans when they thought these might have been lost.

There are many other things that you may be able to give to the parents to help them to remember their baby:

➤ cot cards and wristbands bearing the baby's name and the date and time of birth
➤ a special certificate commemorating the baby's birth
➤ if possible, and with permission from the parents, a tiny lock of hair
➤ cards with images of the baby's handprints and footprints
➤ photographs of the baby, including some taken with the parents and perhaps the wider family.

If you are involved in the delivery of a dead baby, you may be present when the parents take photographs of their baby, or they may ask you to take photographs for them. They may ask you to take a photograph of one of them holding the baby or of a family group. A family group may be the parents and their baby or may, in some cases, involve other family members such as the baby's siblings and grandparents.

I (Ruth) remember being asked, as a junior registrar, to take pictures of a couple as they cradled their stillborn daughter not long after she had been born. None of my clinical teachers had taught me that this was the correct thing to do, but to the parents it seemed the most natural thing in the world and I was encouraged by their behaviour to take part in the process. Looking back on it, I realise I was very privileged to have been involved and the natural manner with which they treated their daughter's body taught me a lot about how to deal with similar cases in the future.

If the parents ask you to help them to take pictures like this, you should agree as long as you feel able. If you find it too sad and strange, ask a senior colleague to help you or ask them to take the pictures instead.

Taking a photograph of a dead baby can be a very difficult and at the same time a profoundly moving thing to do. It would be easy to make the picture look horrible; we have seen many examples of ghastly Polaroid photographs of dead babies. In the past, midwives were often asked to take a photograph of a dead baby so that there was a record in the hospital notes, but this is a task that many will have found appalling and the result would reflect their feelings. It may be that those who have taken ghastly photographs have done so because they would rather be doing anything else. It is possible, with the correct skill, to take a photograph that makes the baby look as though he is asleep rather than dead. It takes special skill to be able to photograph a dead baby in a natural and lifelike way. The work of our mortician colleagues Lee Clarke and Karen Bunce, and of Todd Hochberg,[1] a professional photographer who has an interest in producing beautiful photographs for bereaved families, deserves special mention in this respect.

If your hospital has someone who takes professional quality photographs of this kind, they may be given to the parents as soon as they are printed or left in the mother's hospital notes to be given to her and her partner when they are seen for a follow-up appointment. We have found that whilst some parents are eager to see these pictures and take them home, others will not want to look at them and will be content that they remain in the notes should they want to see them at a later date. It is important that you reassure the parents that you will keep the photographs safely in the notes and that they will be able to look at them or take them home in the future if they wish. We have found that parents may react very differently to the pictures: one parent may want to keep them and cherish them whereas the other may not want to look at them and will want the hospital to keep them, or may only want to look at them once they are alone.

We know that individual responses mean that some women will have pictures on 'public' display in their homes, or even in their workplace, whilst some will have them in their bedroom or another special place away from everyone other than close relations.

MOSES BASKETS AND SMALLER BASKETS

A maternity ward in a unit delivering 3000 to 4000 babies a year needs to have at least two full-sized Moses baskets and a selection of smaller ones, such as the type one would use for a small doll. You may need to be creative about this. We have used baskets that might have been used for bread, which have been transformed by a soft lining and some broderie anglaise trimming. A gynaecology ward should have some tiny ones that in another context would be used for trinkets or keys. All these baskets should have fresh cot linen that is easily washable. Some hospitals have volunteers who will produce tiny knitted or crocheted blankets for dead babies. Lisa's Stars[2] and Upon Butterfly Wings[3] are organisations that have provided us with blankets, bonnets and little pouches for tiny babies. We would also recommend the memory boxes provided by Sands containing hand-knitted blankets in which to wrap the baby, which the parents can then take home, along with other mementoes.

The baby may stay in the room with the parents in the Moses basket for some time, and it is important that she looks as nice as is possible in the circumstances. The basket should ideally be kept in the coolest part of the room, out of direct sunlight, so that the baby does not get too warm. Some parents will ask you to take their baby away for a while; if you put the Moses basket in another room on the ward, make sure everyone on the ward knows that the baby is there so that no one enters the room and finds the dead baby unexpectedly.

The first time I (Ruth) was involved with looking after women with still-births as a junior registrar, I was struck by the senior midwifery sister on the labour ward who would go and find some white flowers (this was in the days when flowers were allowed on hospital wards) and put one in the Moses basket next to the baby with an air of quiet reverence. Flowers are a natural sign of sympathy and commemoration and, by having one or two in the basket, can help us to view the baby with dignity and respect. Parents may want to put little toys in the basket, perhaps a teddy or a doll, or something else that means something special to them and their family. The Sands memory boxes contain two little teddies, the idea being that one can go in the coffin and be buried with the baby and the other can go home with the parents in the box.

SUMMARY: EVERYONE IS DIFFERENT

Everyone will do this kind of thing differently and whilst many parents will look to you for help and guidance, others will have many ideas of their own. Your job, as the health professional, is to help if you can and to stand back and let the parents do what seems right for them in their own way if that is what they prefer. If you feel out of your depth, ask for help from a senior or more experienced colleague.

If you remain open-minded when looking after bereaved parents, you will learn a great deal about how people behave when they are grieving. In the future, you may deal with parents who approach a similar situation in a completely different way, but you will be able to learn something useful from all of them.

REFERENCES

1. www.toddhochberg.com/main.html
2. www.lisasstars.org.uk
3. www.uponbutterflywings.org/

CHAPTER 10

Tests, post-mortems and paperwork

INTRODUCTION

Parents and staff will not usually know the reason for a perinatal death. It is natural for people in this situation to ask for answers. They want to know why the baby died. When parents ask 'Why did our baby die?' they are anxious for an explanation, whilst at the same time worried that the answer will mean that in some way the death was their fault. This chapter examines useful tests to discuss with and offer to the parents when a baby has died.

TESTS ON THE PLACENTA AND UMBILICAL CORD

If there is any suggestion that infection may have played a role in the baby's demise, for example, if the woman had a high temperature or a raised white cell count, or if the liquor had an offensive smell, swabs should be taken from the placenta soon after it is delivered. If the baby is to have a PM, the placenta should be sent fresh, not in formalin, with the baby to the mortuary, and it will be examined along with the baby by the pathologist. If there is to be no PM, the placenta can be sent to the mortuary fixed in formalin to await histological examination. Much useful information can be gleaned from careful examination of the placenta and umbilical cord. In some cases, these findings may explain or confirm the cause of death, with diagnoses such as acute chorioamnionitis, placental infarction, chronic histiocytic intervillositis (CHI) or umbilical hypercoiling.

Acute chorioamnionitis is likely to be found if the cervix has been prematurely dilated or there has been prolonged membrane rupture prior to the delivery. Since these clinical features will hopefully already have been diagnosed, the histological finding of chorioamnionitis serves to confirm what happened and why the pregnancy went wrong rather than to explain it. Often, though, the infection causing the inflammation of chorioamnionitis is not identified by the microbiology laboratory, and the reason for unexpected cervical dilatation or preterm membrane rupture is not elucidated. This can make it difficult to explain the cause of death to parents afterwards: we know *how* the pregnancy went wrong but we do not really know *why.*

Placental infarction in some ways makes more sense as an explanation of pregnancy loss, as it is often seen in the context of a blood clotting disorder or maternal hypertension affecting the placental circulation. It may also be seen with a placental abruption, which may occur spontaneously or in relation to abdominal trauma. All of these conditions may have already been diagnosed clinically, usually before the end of the pregnancy, and histological examination of the placenta confirms what will have already been suspected.

Some more unusual placental conditions, which are not necessarily linked to an antenatal problem, may be diagnosed at PM. One such condition is CHI, which is characterised by an infiltration of the spaces between the placental villi by cells that attack placental cells and cause the deposition of fibrin-like material in place of normal placental tissue. Because the placenta cannot properly function, the condition is associated with severe intrauterine growth restriction and early fetal loss, with few affected pregnancies reaching the late third trimester. The cause of CHI is unclear, although autoimmune factors are thought to be important in some cases.[1] There is a high rate of recurrence: one recent paper has suggested the recurrence rate is 100%.[2] Another study found a higher than usual incidence of fetal congenital malformation associated with CHI[3] and the authors suggest chorionic villous sampling in severely growth-restricted pregnancies. Beyond that, there is currently little useful information about the management of future pregnancies other than monitoring for fetal growth restriction and planning an early delivery if the pregnancy goes beyond 24 weeks.

Umbilical hypercoiling is a condition in which the cord is too tightly twisted, impeding the blood supply along it. Hypercoiled cords have a high umbilical coiling index, defined as greater than 0.3 coils per centimetre, and are associated with fetal growth restriction or sudden IUFD linked to thrombosis in the cord vessels. Interestingly, hypocoiled cords, with a coiling index of less than 0.07 coils per centimetre, are also linked to an increased risk of poor perinatal outcome. It is not clear whether the abnormal coiling is a direct cause of intrauterine pathology or how the abnormal coiling index comes about but finding a hypercoiled cord in an otherwise normal perinatal PM is significant.[4] Careful examination of the umbilical cord after a stillbirth will identify abnormalities in the coiling index that could explain the loss and may help in the planning of future pregnancy care. For example, you can arrange to scan the cord during future pregnancies to see if it is normally coiled and reassure the mother if this is the case. However, ultrasound is an inaccurate predictor of hypercoiling and hypocoiling, either because of observer error or because it seems that the coiling index may change with increasing gestational age.[5]

PERINATAL PM EXAMINATIONS

Parents vary in terms of what tests they want done to try to establish a cause of death. Some will take the view that every test possible should be done, including a PM examination. Others will not want anything that will 'hurt' the baby and will find the thought of their baby's body being cut too awful to consider. Some will want to avoid a PM examination for religious or cultural reasons. Staff should not try to push the parents in one direction or another in regard to this. There is no right answer as to what to do in this situation, but we must be honest about what parents can expect. For example, you should not tell them that a PM will find the answer about why their baby died, as in many cases this will not be true. Some parents will be comforted by the confirmation that there was no known cause of death and that their baby was normal. Some, especially if they have been given unrealistic expectations by staff, will be angry and upset if the examination does not find anything.

We have already stressed the importance of one of the doctors on duty at the time the baby is delivered looking carefully at the baby and documenting the external appearance in the mother's notes. This is especially important in cases where the parents do not wish to have a PM examination.

A PM examination can be carried out on very small babies – say, between 12 and 16 weeks' gestation – but this may not yield any useful information additional to that already seen on an antenatal scan, assuming one was carried out, because the baby is so small. Results will also be very limited in cases where the baby has been dead *in utero* for more than a week and the organs have started to deteriorate. When discussing the pros and cons of a PM, you must be realistic about what the examination may be able to discover and, in some cases, the answer will be 'very little that we didn't already know'. Nonetheless, some parents will be anxious to obtain as much information as possible, so you should be prepared to discuss a PM with them in realistic and sympathetic terms and then to support them in whatever decision they make.

When discussing a PM examination with parents, you must make sure you have enough time to talk it through properly and to answer questions without being interrupted. If you think you may be called away during the discussion, it would be best to mention to the parents that you will be available to discuss things in detail later and simply introduce the subject so that they can think about what they would want to ask and say. Most trusts have leaflets describing perinatal PMs that include frequently asked questions and you can leave one of these with the parents to look at until you are able to give them your full attention.

The rules surrounding consent for perinatal PM came about because of the response of the pathology profession to the scandal at Alder Hey Children's Hospital during the period 1988–1995 when body parts from around 850 babies and children were stored without the knowledge and consent of the parents. Searches at other hospitals revealed that the storage of slides and body parts without parental knowledge or consent was widespread. As a result of these revelations, the current Human Tissue Authority (HTA) and its precise rules about how to obtain consent for a PM examination were established.

The PM consent form is long and detailed, and anyone obtaining consent must have prior training from an HTA-accredited instructor. If you are going to ask for consent for a PM, it is important that you are familiar with the details of the form so that you can go through it methodically with the parents without becoming muddled. It may be best to introduce the main features of the PM and try to find out what the parents think about each section of the form. You will then be able to go through the form checking what they do and do not want. You need to use terminology that the parents will understand: for example, you need to be able to explain what you mean by 'tissue', 'blocks', 'slides' and so on, and be prepared for a lot of questions.

The main points to be discussed are:
➤ what happens in a PM
➤ whether they want a PM
➤ if they do want a PM, whether they want a full one, that will examine all of the body, or they want it to be limited to, say, the heart or the brain
➤ whether they perceive this solely as a way of trying to find out why the baby died or they can also see it as a way of teaching others or providing material for research

➤ the fact that a PM examination will include photographs and may include ultrasound scans and X-rays

➤ whether they agree to tests being carried out to look for bacterial infection, viral infection and the performance of genetic analysis

➤ the fact that the pathologist will examine all of their baby's organs unless the parents say otherwise and that this means removing those organs from the body

➤ the fact that after the organs have been examined, they will be put back into the body cavity, but they will not be arranged as they would have been originally

➤ the fact that the pathologist will make blocks from their baby's body tissues then make slides from those blocks to allow examination of the tissues under the microscope

➤ whether they are prepared to allow the laboratory staff to keep tiny pieces of their baby's body, in the form of blocks and slides, to be used for teaching or research, or whether the staff should dispose of the pieces in a dignified way, or whether they want all of the tiny pieces to go back inside the body at the end of the examination (if this happens, it will be some time, often several weeks, before their baby is available for burial or cremation)

➤ if they do want to have the blocks and slides returned, whether they want them returned with or separately from the body

➤ a report from the pathologist with details of the PM findings can take between 6 and 8 weeks, or however long it takes in your hospital, to be available.

It can take at least half an hour, often longer, to discuss these points and to answer the questions that arise. Once the parents are clear about what they prefer, you can then go through the consent form with them, ticking the relevant boxes and showing them the places where a signature is required. You, as the person taking consent, have to fill in your details on the last page. You must then photocopy the completed consent form and give a copy to the parents.

You do not have to be a doctor to obtain consent for a PM. A nurse or midwife can do this as long as they have had the appropriate training from an HTA-registered instructor.

Perinatal PM examinations should be carried out by specialised perinatal pathologists, and there will not be one available in every hospital. This means that the baby's body will have to be taken to a different hospital for the PM, as is the case at our hospital, and then brought back to the hospital where the baby was delivered after the examination is complete. Careful arrangements need to be made to ensure that the baby is cared for and handled in a dignified fashion on the journeys to and from the PM. These arrangements will usually involve a local funeral director with whom the hospital has a prior agreement or contract. Assuming the baby has to travel for the PM, you should be clear about this when talking to the parents and reassure them that their baby will be treated correctly during the journeys.

If the baby is dressed or wrapped in a shawl in the mortuary, he will remain clothed on the way to the PM examination. Mortuary and laboratory staff should ensure that he is dressed in the same way when he returns.

It is useful for parents to have a discussion with one of the morticians about how their baby will look after the PM. The baby's body cavity will be sewn up and his skull will have been cut to allow examination of the brain and then put back into place. Parents will always have the option to see their baby after the PM and it is possible to disguise the scars with hats and other clothes.

TESTS FOR THE MOTHER

The main tests to carry out on the mother after a perinatal death are blood tests for a thrombophilia screen and an anti-cardiolipin antibody (ACA) screen to look for anti-phospholipid syndrome (APS). Both are related to an increased tendency for blood-clot formation and are linked to recurrent pregnancy loss. They may not have been suspected prior to the pregnancy problems and may only come to light as a result of testing after a pregnancy loss. The results may vary from pregnancy to pregnancy and some women with these conditions have losses as well as successful pregnancies.

There are several versions of thrombophilia: all involve the patient having an increased tendency to form blood clots, which may arise from different parts of the coagulation cascade being abnormal. There can be deficiencies in natural anticoagulants including protein C, protein S and anti-thrombin III, or there may be a gene mutation such as factor V Leiden.

APS is an autoimmune condition in which blood will clot more easily than usual. This occurs because of the formation of antibodies against phospholipids in cell membranes, provoking clots to form in blood vessels. APS may be primary, when the woman has no other related conditions, or secondary, when there are other autoimmune diseases such as systemic lupus erythematosus.

The thrombophilia screen requires four coagulation screen bottles and the ACA screen requires two bottles of clotted blood.

The tests may need to be repeated 3 months later, as there may be some fluctuation in results associated with the recent pregnancy. This can be arranged at the follow-up appointment.

Other tests may be warranted depending on the clinical situation. For example, a woman complaining of flu-like symptoms prior to a second trimester loss may have contracted listeria, and if she is still feverish she should have blood cultures examined.

Tests for diabetes and thyroid dysfunction are often carried out after a perinatal loss but are not necessary. Neither well-controlled diabetes nor treated thyroid dysfunction are risk factors for recurrent pregnancy loss.[6]

CERTIFICATION ABOUT STILLBIRTH AND NEONATAL DEATH

A stillbirth certificate is a legal requirement for any baby born after 24 completed weeks of pregnancy who showed no signs of life. A baby born at any gestation that showed signs of life at birth and then died will need a birth certificate and a death certificate.

If a doctor is to sign a stillbirth certificate, he or she must have seen the baby's body. This might have been on the ward or in the mortuary. If a doctor was present when the dead baby was delivered, he or she should complete and sign a stillbirth certificate before going off duty, as this then prevents any delay for the parents. It will be easier for them if they can have the certificate quickly, certainly before they want to go home, rather than having to wait for someone else to go down to the mortuary and see the baby's body before signing the certificate, or worse, having to come back to the hospital to collect the certificate.

The stillbirth certificate is required so that the stillbirth can be registered at the registry office, which allows the body to be released by the mortuary for burial or cremation. It may be easier for parents if someone at the hospital gives the stillbirth certificate to the local registrar rather than giving the certificate to the parents and leaving them with the responsibility of taking it to the registry office. The mother (or father if the parents are married) must still register the stillbirth before a burial or cremation. There is a 3-month limit after which the baby cannot be registered, but in this case, the registry office, providing they had the stillbirth certificate, could then issue a certificate of disposal that would enable a funeral to take place. If the original stillbirth certificate is not available, a duplicate can be produced by the hospital, thus enabling the registry office to provide a certificate of disposal.

To sign a death certificate in the event of a neonatal death, a doctor will have ideally seen the baby alive and then dead. This is relatively straightforward if the baby was admitted to the neonatal unit and then died, but it can be more problematic if the baby died on the labour ward very soon after delivery. If a baby of, say, 22 weeks' gestation, is delivered and shows signs of life, but is too small to be resuscitated and ventilated and dies within an hour or so, this should be registered as a neonatal death. Therefore, it is good practice for midwives to call a doctor when someone is delivering at 20 weeks' gestation or more, so that the doctor can be present at the delivery and witness whether the baby shows signs of life. The doctor can then document clearly in the mother's notes what they have seen and complete the relevant certificate without delay. However, this is not always practical, so if a doctor was not present at the birth, he or she can then take the word of the parents and midwife that the baby showed signs of life and then died and sign the death certificate. This will be accepted by staff in the registry office and by coroners. In the past, this was not common practice and we have known of cases in which parents and midwives have witnessed signs of life in a very small baby who was pre-viable then, because no doctor was present, there was confusion regarding which type of certificate to issue. The resulting delays meant that the baby could not be registered and the body not released for burial. In one of the cases known to us, it was only the intervention of the local coroner that allowed the situation to be resolved and a certificate issued long after the event. This kind of administrative difficulty was harrowing for the parents and can now be avoided.

SUMMARY

Investigations are vital to try to find out why a baby died. If you are organising tests in these circumstances, you need to be able to communicate clearly what is involved and why they are recommended. Attention to detail with the necessary certification can smooth the path for bereaved parents, and a clear knowledge of relevant test results can help enormously with perinatal loss counselling and planning for future pregnancies.

REFERENCES

1. Boyd TK, Redline RW. Chronic histiocytic intervillositis: a placental lesion associated with recurrent reproductive loss. *Hum Pathol*. 2000; **31**(11): 1389–96.
2. Parant O, Capdet J, Kessler S et al. Chronic intervillositis of unknown etiology (CIUE): relation between placental lesions and perinatal outcome. *Eur J Obstet Gynecol Reprod Biol*. 2009; **143**(1): 9–13.
3. Rota C, Carles D, Schaeffer V et al. Pronostic périnatal des grossesses compliquées d'intervillites chroniques placentaires [Perinatal prognosis of pregnancies complicated by placental chronic intervillitis]. *J Gynecol Obstet Biol Reprod (Paris)*. 2006; **35**(7): 711–19.

4. de Laat MW, Franx A, van Alderen ED *et al*. The umbilical coiling index: a review of the literature. *J Matern Fetal Neonatal Med*. 2005; **17**(2): 93–100.

5. Predanic M, Perni SC, Chasen ST *et al*. Assessment of umbilical cord coiling during the routine fetal sonographic anatomic survey in the second trimester. *J Ultrasound Med*. 2005; **24**(2): 185–91.

6. RCOG. *The Investigation and Treatment of Couples with Recurrent Miscarriage*. Green-top guideline 17. London: RCOG; 2011. Available at: www.rcog.org.uk/files/rcog-corp/GTG17recurrentmiscarriage.pdf (accessed 17 August 2012).

CHAPTER 11

Funeral arrangements, including burial and cremation

INTRODUCTION

This chapter is about what happens when the mother is discharged from hospital and what follows regarding funeral arrangements.

At the beginning of the book, we discussed our reasons for not being culturally specific, but when it comes to burial or cremation it is essential that the parents' culture be taken into account. Beliefs and preferences about the handling of a dead body and its disposal vary between different religions and it is important that staff find out if the parents have any particular preferences. Muslims and Jews will not want a PM examination and will want a burial rather than a cremation. Hindus and Sikhs will want a burial for a dead baby, although adults will traditionally be cremated. Having said this, it is important not to make assumptions about what parents want and to check before making any arrangements. There still needs to be an individual person-centred approach, but it will help parents if the staff they deal with are culturally aware.

If a baby dies before 24 weeks' gestation, there is no official recognition that the baby existed and there is no legal requirement for a formal burial or cremation. Most hospitals have some sort of certificate or memorial card to commemorate the death of a baby before 24 weeks, and parents find it helpful to have their loss acknowledged in this way. Some, but not all, hospitals make arrangements for pre-viable babies to have a burial or cremation, and there will be a form to complete so that parents can say which they would prefer and how much they would like to be involved.

The fact that no formal record of birth or death is recorded can be difficult for parents and it is essential that medical staff do not necessarily make distinctions based on this legal definition. The death of a baby needs to be given the same significance by staff as by the parents. Hospital staff need to be prepared to help parents make arrangements for the burial or cremation of babies who are born prior to 24 weeks' gestation.

Some parents ask to take the remains of their early pregnancy home so that they can, for instance, bury them in the garden and plant a rose bush or some other flower as a memorial. This can be the case after terminations for fetal abnormality as well as after miscarriages. Some staff find this idea strange, especially after a termination; if you do, it is important that your attitude is not conveyed to the parents.

After 24 weeks' gestation or a live birth at any gestation, there is a legal requirement that the birth and death are registered at a registry office. All deaths after 24 weeks are registered, but births are only registered if the baby was born alive. The Sands publication *Pregnancy Loss and the Death of a Baby: guidelines for professionals*[1] does a superb job describing the intricacies of registration. Medical staff need to recognise that parents may well need help or guidance to do this; it is likely to be their first time registering a death. Within the hospital, there needs to be someone whose role includes being responsible for supporting parents through the next steps that they need to take. It is not enough to have helped someone through all the hurdles of giving birth then abandon them once they leave hospital.

LEAVING THE BABY IN THE MORTUARY

If parents are leaving their baby behind them when they are discharged from hospital, the care of their baby will be of paramount importance to most of them. They need to know where she is going and who will be looking after her. Hospital staff need to make it as easy as possible for parents to visit their baby in the mortuary. Some mothers and members of her family make numerous visits, whilst others will not feel the need to go at all or will only go once or twice. Therefore, it behoves you to be familiar with the mortuary and to be able to describe it to the parents if this will help. When we provided pregnancy-loss training for staff, we initially had the mortician come and talk to the group but realised that it was much better for the staff to go to the mortuary. The thought of doing this actually often frightened them. It was only by going, seeing and experiencing the mortuary and how it was set up, especially from a parent's point of view, that they were able to be less fearful. If we had not challenged these fears then staff would have passed on something of their anxiety (consciously or unconsciously) to bereaved mothers and their families. We are fortunate that the mortuary in the hospital where we work is not in the basement. Staff who have worked in institutions where it has been, have described their feelings of fear associated with going to the 'bowels' of the hospital; an area without natural light could bring up thoughts of dread associated with their feelings about death. Even more fortuitous for us, and especially so for parents, we have two morticians who take their work in caring for the babies of bereaved mothers and fathers very seriously indeed.

If the baby has to go to another venue for the PM, it is important that parents are informed about when their baby has gone and when he has returned. They need to be able to locate in their minds where he is at any one time. Following a PM, the mortuary staff will need to be even more sensitive as to how they present the baby to his relatives. It is possible to arrange him in such a way that his parents and other family members will not be able to see the effects of him having been cut open. After the PM, one woman, not at our hospital thankfully, had not been given any information as to what to expect. Unfortunately, her baby was not dressed adequately enough and she saw, in her words, 'the very crude stitching' of her baby daughter's abdomen. This caused her a lot of pain and it was a memory that stayed with her for a long time.

TAKING THE BABY HOME

A baby will remain at the mortuary until the funeral, unless the parents wish to take their baby home. In our experience this is unusual, but for the few who do, it is normal and understandable. Parents will say that they wanted to have their baby daughter home with them for a night before she was buried, or that they wanted to have her with them in their garden or some other place that is special to them. Again, even though some members of staff may recoil from the idea of taking a dead baby home, they should treat the parents with professionalism and understanding and not upset them further by showing their feelings. The media storm that surrounded United States Republican candidate Rick Santorum when he talked about how he and his wife had taken home their son Gabriel, who died shortly after being born very prematurely, to meet their other children, shows how difficult this subject is for many people.[2] Whilst most commentators expressed sympathy for the Santorum family because of their sad loss, many were openly hostile and regarded what they had done as 'weird' and 'bizarre'.

There is absolutely no reason why a parent or a couple cannot take their dead baby home with them when they are discharged. It is important to emphasise this fact, as many medical personnel think that there are legal or ethical reasons against this. The baby belongs to her parents and no one else; it is not kidnapping or illegal. No one would dream of preventing a live baby from going home unless there were safeguarding issues. As not many people choose to take a dead baby home, we wonder if staff members' inhibitions mean that they do not know it is a possibility, so they do not discuss this option with parents. In many cultures and religions, it is traditional to have the person who has died at home with them prior to the funeral. It can be a meaningful way of honouring the life of that person and a way of acknowledging the reality of their death. If it was a more acceptable notion to medical personnel that parents leave the hospital with their dead baby, more may well choose to do so. Hospital staff could make arrangements with the parents as to what they wanted to do regarding the funeral; it may be that the baby stays at home for a limited time and comes back to the hospital mortuary or it may be that the parents arrange a funeral and the funeral directors look after the baby.

If you find this a difficult concept, it might help you to talk to someone who is not afraid of these ideas or to attend training that will help you be more confident.

FUNERALS, BURIALS AND CREMATIONS

All hospitals need appropriate staff to be involved in creating policies that deal with the sensitive disposal of all babies, regardless of gestation. We have been part of a multi-disciplinary pregnancy-loss working party at our hospital for several years. The specific aim of the working party has been to look at the complex matters concerning pregnancy loss. The working party has managed to be instrumental in improving the care families receive. Some of the work we have done has been to improve the hospital's management of funerals, burials and cremations. We have come to realise how significant a loss at any gestation can be and we have created policies and procedures to acknowledge this. We have outlined below some of what we have learnt.

Funerals for early losses

Because staff noticed what women and their partners go through at the time of a loss and their concerns as to what happens to their baby, we arranged that when a woman has an early loss, careful examination is made of the remains of the pregnancy in the histology laboratory. If there is a recognisable baby or baby parts, these remains are sent to the mortuary. By 'recognisable', we mean to the naked eye, either through miscarriage or ectopic pregnancy, for example, whether delivered naturally or by surgery. We have known there to be recognisable tiny intact fetuses as early as at 7 weeks' gestation. Ideally, the woman will have been told in advance by staff that this is what will happen. In practice, staff find this a difficult aspect of care to discuss, either because of the perceived delicacy of the matter or because staff change and are not aware of the hospital's protocols, but it is essential that parents are informed. Staff must ensure they have all the information necessary to make sure they are involved in making choices. This includes mentioning the policy when consent is taken prior to an ERPC or surgical removal of an ectopic pregnancy.

When a recognisable baby or baby parts are found, the mother and her partner are offered a burial or cremation, which will be arranged by the hospital morticians and chaplains. It is important to remember that the parents have the first option to arrange something themselves, but, in our experience, the majority opt for the hospital to make the arrangements on their behalf. We have negotiated burial and cremation services with the local authority so that each baby or the baby parts will be in an individual coffin and, in the case of cremation, the baby is cremated individually. The hospital has a contract with a local funeral director. They take responsibility for arranging transport of the coffins from the hospital to the crematorium or the cemetery. We have two sizes of coffins; one for smaller babies or baby remains and the other for bigger babies. The ones we currently use are white, lined with satin-type material and have enough room in them for parents to put in a small soft toy and other significant mementoes. The cremated remains are then available for collection from the crematorium.

We are honest when talking to mothers and their partners, and in our leaflets, that the cremated remains when the baby is of an early gestation mostly come from the coffin. This does not seem to matter at all because within the ashes are the remnants of their baby. If parents opt to collect the ashes, there are many creative ways of using them to commemorate their baby. Many people opt to scatter the ashes in meaningful places; others bury them in a pot together with a plant (so that if they move house they can still take them) or directly into the ground in their garden in a spot that means something to them. Alternatively, they are kept together with other mementoes. If mothers do not want to collect the cremated remains, then they are scattered by crematorium staff in an area that is specially designated for babies and children.

The alternative to cremation is burial. Burial means that the baby is buried in a shared grave with other babies in one of the local cemeteries. Some parents find it a comfort that their baby will not be alone, whilst others do not feel it is right. Those parents who do not want a shared grave can purchase an individual plot for their baby. The shared graves are in an area designated for babies and children. The local authority ensures that the grave is securely covered until such time as the required number of babies is buried (usually 14 babies are buried together if they are less than 24 weeks' gestation, and four if they are over 24 weeks or if they are neonatal deaths); the grave is then permanently grassed over. They also provide a headstone that acknowledges the babies within the grave who have died between the dates the graves opened and closed. This was a joint venture between the hospital and the borough, with the borough providing the headstones and the hospital paying for the lettering. We decided against individual names in the interests of confidentiality and not wanting to cause additional pain. Mothers and fathers can negotiate with the borough about putting a permanent marker on the shared grave for their individual baby.

Whether parents choose a burial or cremation, one of the hospital's chaplains will conduct a short individual funeral service. The chaplains devise funeral services for those with or without a Christian belief. Other religious leaders are available for people of other faiths. We have a slot of half an hour at the crematorium and this allows for up to three babies to be commemorated. When we started to provide funeral services, we envisaged that they would be shared services for a number of families, but we quickly realised that it was better to give each baby an individual time. This was mainly due to the fact that the circumstances of each baby's death almost always varied and that it was not possible to honour them collectively in an appropriate manner. One of the morticians and the chaplain are present at the crematorium to greet those attending the funeral and to help ensure the service goes well. Many of the parents will have met the morticians previously, either when they visited their baby or when they have dropped off something they want to be put in their baby's coffin. For each individual baby there is a printed service sheet; not all parents give their baby a first name, but this is included if they do. If the parents have negotiated in advance with the chaplains, meaningful prayers, poems or prose are included together with their choice of a piece of music. If they have not made contact, then the chaplains use their experience to provide meaningful words and music. Each individual service does not last more than 10 minutes. Whilst this may seem short, in actuality it gives enough time to honour the existence of the baby and the significance of the loss.

Not all parents attend the service, but most of them appreciate that the hospital provides this facility. Individual families do different things regarding the funeral; sometimes just the mother attends, or a select group, or lots of extended family members come with the parents. We have been encouraged that at the follow-up perinatal loss clinic patients report that, despite it being a hugely painful thing to have to do, they are appreciative of the opportunity to attend a funeral service and having the choice to bury or cremate their baby. They describe the funeral service as being worthwhile and a form of closure.

When there is no recognisable baby or baby parts found during the examination in the histology department, we have arranged with the local crematorium that they take responsibility for the sensitive disposal of these remains. Previously, they were treated as clinical waste. We realised that treating unrecognisable remains in this way did not give the loss the dignity it required. Since we have found that gestations of as little as 7 weeks are sometimes recognisable and, equally, that later losses are not, we needed to be able to comfort those parents without recognisable remains with the knowledge that their baby will be given as much respect as possible. Unfortunately, there is no way we can provide a funeral service for parents when there are no recognisable remains.

Funerals for later losses

If a baby of any gestation has lived and subsequently died or has died after 24 completed weeks of gestation, then there is a legal requirement for registration. However, there is no legal requirement that the family has to arrange the funeral, but, in our experience, parents tend to organise their own funeral and staff within the hospital need to be prepared to support them in this difficult task. If mothers or couples want the hospital to do so, we will still make the arrangements on their behalf. This means that the funeral directors who have the hospital contract will make the arrangements and will negotiate a suitable time for the service with the parents. Very occasionally, making funeral arrangements for their baby is too much for parents. If this is the case, we have devised a system in which parents give their written consent to allow arrangements be made on their behalf. For some, that is the end of their involvement; they do not want to know when the service will take place. Others will want to know and attend the service, even if they were unable to deal with making the arrangements.

SUMMARY

The funeral, burial or cremation of a baby who has died is the last tangible thing in which parents can be involved. It is important for hospital staff to enable them to be as involved as they wish. It is the final act of giving dignity and worth to a loved and desired baby who has died.

REFERENCES

1. Schott J, Henley A, Kohner N. *Pregnancy Loss and the Death of a Baby: guidelines for professionals.* 3rd ed. London: Sands; 2007.
2. Donaldson James S. *Experts: Rick Santorum grief is typical, but taking body home, unusual.* New York, NY: ABC News; 6 January 2012. Available at: http://abcnews.go.com/Health/ rick-santorum-dead-baby-critics-lambasted-families-grieve/story?id=15306750#. T6tXkFJ62S (accessed 17 August 2012).

CHAPTER 12

Support for parents after the death and the longer lasting effects of grief

INTRODUCTION

This chapter is an attempt to describe our experience of working with grieving women and their partners in the aftermath of the diagnosis and the delivery of their dead baby.

The impact of a baby dying can be huge on parents, their families and friends. It can feel to them as if they are living in a completely different place from people who have not experienced such a loss. Following the death of their baby, they may not be able to understand why people in the old place still carry on as if nothing of any note has happened.

The theories about grief are changing; the expectation used to be that people would go through certain stages of grief and then move on, having left their relationship to the deceased behind. It was thought that grief was a bit like an illness, and if people were given the right treatment or did the correct exercise then they would get better and recover. It is now recognised that people will experience grief and mourning, but, rather than moving on, they will create a 'continuing bond' with the person who has died.

> One sees that grief is never finished, that the way the bereaved relate to the deceased changes as they develop over the life cycle, whether they be young or old mourners. Yet there seems to be a lack of appropriate language for describing mourning as part of the life cycle. People need to stop thinking of grief as

being entirely present or absent. People rarely just do not 'get over it', nor do they ever really find 'closure'. The phrase 'continuing bonds' is one contribution to a new language that reflects a new understanding of this process.[1]

As well as being extremely useful for parents who have had a baby die, this acknowledgement of continuing bonds is also challenging. There are fewer tangible bonds with a baby who has died either in the womb or shortly after birth than with someone who has lived their whole life. However, the dreams of the life the baby would have had and the life that the parents, family and wider society would have had with the baby can become part of the bonds. It is really important that mothers, fathers and others are allowed to talk about their connection with their baby and also the loss of the future they envisaged.

As they go through the months of their bereavement, many women talk about how they imagine the stages of development their baby would be going through. For example, 'she would be smiling by this stage'; 'he would be crawling now'. We know of one woman who actually visited a nursery next door to where she was working because she needed to know where her son would have been if he had lived. It can be beneficial to ask bereaved parents if their baby resembled either of them or any one in their family. We have seen babies as young as 20 weeks' gestation who look like one or both of their parents. Not all, but many parents welcome an opportunity to show you photographs of their baby. This can be very permission-giving for them and you are contributing to their creation of continuing bonds.

> Bereavement does not go away but is a difficult and expected part of the normal life cycle; it is a period of loss, of change and transition in how the bereaved relate to themselves, to the deceased, and to the world around them. A continuing bond does not mean, however, that people live in the past. The very nature of mourners' daily lives is changed by the death. The deceased are both present and absent. One cannot ignore this fact and the tension this creates in the bereavement process. Connections to the dead need to be legitimized. People need to talk about the deceased, to participate in memorial rituals, and to understand that their mourning is an evolving, not a static, process. In the words of a nineteenth-century rabbi, Samuel David Luzzatto, 'Memory sustains man in the world of life'.[1]

THE EXPERIENCE OF GRIEF

Initially, grief completely fills up the existence of the bereaved parents and often they anticipate that eventually it will diminish. By cooperating with their mourning, they realise that their grief remains the same, but what happens is that, in time, their capacity for life expands. Gradually, as people grieve, they come to understand that they have more capacity for their physical, emotional and mental energy and, as described, they have more ability to include new things in life or to resume aspects of their previous life.

The first few weeks following the death of a baby are often very busy and active from a practical point of view, and it can be somewhat of a relief that these come to an end with the funeral. That said, people can feel empty because there is nothing more that can be done for their baby. It can be at this point that the reality of what their baby dying means begins to hit mothers and fathers. On that note, it helps to remember that women and men may well grieve differently. For example, when the loss has occurred at an early stage of pregnancy, the father may not experience the loss as significantly as the mother. When talking to Salvation Army captains on placement with the hospital chaplains, one man explained that he thought of himself as having two children whereas his wife always said that she had three but that one had miscarried. Another example is that of an older woman who had an early miscarriage and who found it very painful that her husband did not acknowledge that she had lost a baby and that this was a significant loss for her. She pointed out the discrepancy in his thinking by adding that had she wanted to terminate the pregnancy he would have recognised the baby as being real and would have accused her of killing it. These two situations illustrate some of the differences felt by men and women.

Sometimes for a man, the loss and the grief are not so much for his baby but for the change in his partner. His experience of the woman's grief means that he is not able to understand or share that loss and he wants his 'old' partner back. This difference in the way they grieve can be tricky for both partners, as the woman may be puzzled as to why her man does not relate to her loss in a similar way to herself and the man may think she is being self-indulgent. Conversely, we have met many men who feel that they are sidelined and that their loss is not given much credence, as all the focus is on their partners. The Child Bereavement Charity information sheet[2] regarding different ways of grieving makes the essential point that even if there is a sense of shared grief, mourning for a profound loss is solitary. Individuals react to grief in their own individual way and it is important to have no preconceptions as to how anyone should react.

The reason grief is difficult for most of us is because it hurts and it hurts *so* much. Grief is such an intense pain. There are many words used to describe grief but not many can really convey the depth of feeling that accompanies the journey that the death of a baby evokes. Not only has a mother to give birth to her baby who has died but also to give birth to her grief.

Having worked with many grieving individuals, we suggest that we all have an in-built capacity to grieve and if we can cooperate with it and get help when required, we do eventually come through the pain. Many people struggle with this and feel they should not be feeling as they do (sad, confused, bereft etc.) or for as long as they do. We live in a culture that rewards both sexes for being strong and coping. 'You are really strong' is often said to parents if they are not visibly upset in front of others. This can add to the pressure of grieving for both a mother and a father as the subtle, or not so subtle, message is that if they are outwardly upset they are being weak. This is not the case: to allow the pain of bereavement requires a lot of strength. Grieving is very demanding.

For many people, the death of a baby may be their first experience of a significant person dying and therefore their initial encounter with grief. Obviously, others will have had previous experience of grieving, but there is something unique about a baby dying. The baby and mother have been together from conception and the baby has had no life beyond that contained in its mother's womb; you cannot get closer than that. So grieving is new for many parents and they do not know what to expect.

Grief has physical, emotional and mental components. Feeling physically and mentally exhausted is common. People often report an inability to sleep and concentrate for any length of time. Sometimes, an inability to get to sleep or waking in the middle of the night and then not being able to get back to sleep, is due to the fact that people, either consciously or unconsciously, avoid thinking or feeling during the day. Therefore, the only time that they have to address their grief is when they settle down for the night or when they have had some sleep but wake up and stay awake. It can be useful for people to write down the thoughts and feelings that are preventing them from sleeping at the time, as it is a way of acknowledging important information and also a way of clearing their mind so that they can have rest. These written observations are often beneficial and can be looked at in the daytime and acted upon if necessary.

Grief can also manifest itself as a loss of appetite and a general disinterest in anything around you. When you are grieving, there is a limited amount of energy available for anything other than experiencing and managing the loss. Because mourning demands a lot of strength, it may be necessary to take time away from the world.

Anger is a recognised aspect of grief and one way it manifests is that bereaved mothers will become intolerant of other mothers' inadequate parenting. They will see women shouting at their children in the street and this evokes a feeling of unfairness, as they anticipate that they would never treat children in that way. In our experience, very few women express anger towards the baby that died. They do not seem to blame the baby for not surviving or for not trying harder to live. It is only occasionally that women will express this kind of frustration towards their dead son or daughter.

Another way anger can be present is if the parents have not been cared for in the hospital. We cannot emphasise enough the impact inadequate care has on grieving parents. All too often we hear mothers and fathers and their families express how they could manage their baby's death 'if only' everything had been done properly. The experience of inadequate care interferes with their ability to grieve. Where there is evidence of inadequate care, it may be really important for parents to make formal complaints and even sue the hospital. They should be supported by staff in taking these kinds of actions. However, if they only focus on those angry feelings then their ability to grieve will be delayed. Anyone working with couples and families in this situation needs to assist them gently in the dual tasks of trying to get the hospital to make reparation and managing the actual death of their baby, whatever the cause.

Coming to terms with the death and the loss of a baby is hugely demanding and so many changes happen that are beyond the individual's control. In the early days, people are aware of the physical death and the separation from their baby. Many women find it difficult that their body heals very quickly after the birth. We have known women who are reluctant to lose their pregnancy weight, as it would be too painful to be without something related to their baby. The return of monthly periods is also often difficult, a painful reminder and obvious evidence that they are no longer pregnant. This is not about women being in denial about the fact that their baby has died; it is the difference between what they know intellectually and how the reality of their loss is experienced. As mothers and fathers gradually adjust to their baby's death, they begin to understand that they have to grieve for the loss of their dreams. Dreams of how their baby would have been; what their baby would have been doing; how they would look; how they will never crawl, walk, talk or play football and so on. This loss can be profound; as we said earlier, almost from the beginning of a pregnancy, parents-to-be invest a huge amount in the fledging baby and their future with that baby.

There is a particular strangeness for women whose babies die before their due date. Many women know scan dates and appointments with midwives and doctors in advance and when these dates approach they are yet another reminder of what should be happening and is not. The estimated due date is also challenging; it is often dreaded and feared. In actuality, the day itself often does not seem to be as bad as anticipated. Our observations would be that it is helpful for mothers and fathers to mark the day as being something special. One couple we know started a collection of stones from the special places that they visited on the anniversary of their baby's due date. For some women it is a relief once the due date is passed; for others it means that their grieving moves on to the fact that they would no longer be pregnant but should have had their baby with them. GP colleagues have told us that women have presented themselves at the surgery with odd pains or vague symptoms of being unwell, only for it to become apparent that their baby would have been due that day. One GP we know marks the due date in a patient's notes if she miscarries, so that she is forewarned when the patient turns up in the surgery in this way.

ANNIVERSARIES

The problem with dates is that they come around every year and it is likely that the significant dates in the year of the baby's death will remain so every year. Some parents find it easier when they are able to say that their baby died last year: it gives some sense of distance and some solace that they have survived a calendar year. Other anniversaries and dates that at first glance seem not to be connected with the death of the baby may take on a different meaning; for example, the parents' birthdays are different because their baby is not there.

One day that is challenging for bereaved mothers is Mother's Day. It is often dreaded; if there are no other children, the bereaved mother will wonder if anyone remembers that she, too, is a mother and just because she does not have her baby with her it is her day too. She will be comforted if other family members get her a Mother's Day card or something else to show that she is remembered as a mother. Mother's Day for a woman who has live children can also be tough, as she will want to celebrate feeling special with those children. However, it is important to remember that on each Mother's Day she is highly likely initially to be very aware of the absence of the baby, and later the child, that is missing. Father's Day is also an annual event that will present a challenge for fathers in very similar ways. Obviously, Christmas, Easter and other holidays need to be carefully thought about as to how they will be managed.

As human beings, we like to feel that we have control over life. For some this is highly likely to be an unconscious attitude. The death of a baby brings the realisation that we do not have as much power as we would like. One of the consequences of the disturbance caused by a baby dying manifests for some people in their worrying about something dreadful happening to their remaining significant others. For example, they may not like their partners or other children to be away from them. They imagine car accidents and other terrible catastrophes occurring when they are apart. This is likely to be a temporary fear, and it can be helped by the significant others reassuring them by telephoning to let them know they are okay. When people's abilities to cope have been stretched beyond capacity, they do not need any further stretching. This is why women and their partners need to know that they will have consistent and continuing support in a future pregnancy. They need a sense of being held by the caregivers with whom they will be involved.

Another perplexing attribute of grief is that it is not consistent or predictable. It is not possible to predict in advance how you will feel, so it is useful for bereaved people to be flexible when making plans. We often suggest that any plans have a proviso that includes something like 'I will if I can, but I only know how I am feeling from moment to moment.' Bereaved parents sometimes find that the events they dread are the ones they manage quite well and other ones they think will be easy they find unbearable. A simple trip to the bakers turns into a nightmare when you bump into a member of the antenatal group with her baby. Going to a family wedding or christening can be dreaded but may turn out not to be as difficult as had been anticipated. Bereaved parents can do nothing about this except to adopt an attitude of kindness towards themselves and each other and be patient regarding their own or other peoples' expectations.

There can be such a strong desire to return to normal that the experience of grief is at times resented. Grieving parents, particularly mothers, often feel bitter about other people's apparent ability to return to normal after their baby's death. It does not appear to take long for people to stop asking how she is feeling or acknowledging her baby and her loss. It is not uncommon for women to state that they feel that other people have forgotten and that they and the world have moved on whilst they cannot. It is difficult for grieving mothers to understand that they are sometimes the ones who have to educate others as to how they want to be treated. They can be resentful that it is yet another thing they have to do on top of their grief. In truth, it is problematic for others to know how to talk about a baby's death once the events surrounding the death are completed. People are scared of hurting the mother or opening her wounds, so they stop asking how she and her partner are feeling. This sometimes hurts tremendously. Other people seem to be prying or want to tell the bereaved mother and father how they should be feeling. Because the death itself is so wrong, it is hard for people to get it right all of the time.

THE FOLLOW-UP APPOINTMENT

One of the main things people want to know following the death of their baby is why it happened. At the hospital where we work, we offer parents an appointment to come back and discuss the outcome of the tests or PM with a consultant obstetrician and a women's health counsellor. We have found that is really useful to have people from the two different professions who can care for the parents and any other family member who attends, as together we are likely to be able to cover all the aspects of their loss. Due to the length of time it takes to get a PM report, the appointments occur approximately 8 weeks following the death. This can sometimes feel like an appalling length of time to wait, but we have found that people's ability to make full use of the appointment is impaired if the meeting is too close to the actual time of the death. This appointment takes place in the hospital away from the areas where women attended clinics when they were pregnant or where they gave birth. We recognise that coming back to the hospital can be painful and the sight of other pregnant women in an antenatal clinic also sometimes causes anguish. This is why these appointments take place elsewhere. The purpose of the appointment is to give parents the results of the investigations, to talk about their experience of their pregnancy and the death of the baby, and the care they received. It is also an opportunity to check on how they are managing their grief. Additionally, it gives parents an opportunity to discuss any concerns they have regarding another pregnancy and how they will be looked after in future. It is important to have this discussion when patients are ready for it and it may be that in the future they will want a pre-conception discussion in order for them to feel as confident as they can before embarking on the scary journey of another pregnancy. The consultant obstetrician will usually write a letter for the patient following this appointment outlining the discussion regarding the cause of death and recommendations for how she should be looked after in any future pregnancy. A copy of this letter is also sent to her GP.

There is no timescale for how long an individual's grief will last. How the grief manifests and how individuals manage their grief will vary. We have known bereaved mothers who, as a way of coping, resume work and their previous lifestyle very quickly. To adjust to the enormity of what has happened, other people need to take their time and, for example, have a year off work. It is essential that nobody decides what the length of time of intense grieving or time away from normal duties should be for any mother or father.

GOING BACK TO WORK

Returning to work is a significant event. When women are absent from work, they have power over their environment to some extent. They can decide whether to venture out; to avoid pregnant women; to turn back and go home if they are vulnerable by being in the outside world. Returning to their job means that they have to be ready to give up this level of control. We have noticed that it is such a different experience for women if they have been in charge of deciding when they return to work. Women who want to go back to work because they are ready or because they have become bored at home are in a very different position from those who feel pressured to resume work. This pressure can be internal or external. For example, we have known women who either felt obliged to go back to work or were hassled into returning to their jobs who have had to go on sick leave again.

Going back to work is full of meaning. It is making a statement to the wider world that you are coping; that you are able to manage everyday life. Additionally, functioning at work usually requires concentration, the ability to negotiate with colleagues and so on; as we have indicated, grief has temporarily robbed individuals of most of these abilities. As well as fulfilling the requirements of the job, many women have to deal with colleagues either being or becoming pregnant. This will be a challenge: a woman in this position will not be unhappy for her colleague or wish her to have a pregnancy loss, but she will have to manage the loneliness of her loss again.

There may be people who last saw her when she was pregnant and who will be unaware of the death of the baby. These people ask excitedly 'How is the baby?' and are devastated when they are told that the baby has died. The enquirer feels wrong and embarrassed and the mother can feel exposed.

Many women go back to their jobs at the time when they would have been leaving to go on maternity leave. This is actually a psychologically difficult thing to do and another part of the loss of their dreams. Women who do not particularly like their job have often looked forward to a year off work with their baby.

Many bosses are unfamiliar with how to manage the return to work of a bereaved mother; therefore, unless managers or human resource departments educate themselves, they can cause more damage and hurt. One woman asked if an email could be sent to her colleagues explaining that she was returning to work after the death of her full-term baby. She wanted to try to ensure she would avoid any of the embarrassment we have described above. She also wanted co-workers to know that it was all right with her if people talked to her about her daughter – in fact, this is what she wanted. Her personnel managers refused her request, as they thought some of her colleagues might be upset! This insensitive refusal caused her to feel hurt, angry and increased her sense of isolation. She understandably felt she was being asked to bear the burden of other people's inability to deal with her situation. The Sands organisation has recently produced leaflets called *Returning to Work after the Death of Your Baby* and *Information for Employers: helping a bereaved parent return to work*. These give very good advice to both parties. The information in these leaflets can be used to help avoid similar situations. Interestingly, one of the suggestions is sending an email to staff to help smooth the return.

GPs and other health professionals can be essential in supporting grieving women and their families. It is important to remember that however long the active period of grief is, it is likely to be temporary. GPs can help enormously by providing sick notes until such time as the woman herself indicates that she is ready to go back. In our experience, very few women use their grief as a way of skiving.

Legally, a baby does not exist until 24 weeks' gestation and when there is a death at that or a later gestation, a woman is entitled to maternity leave. This can be very frustrating for women who feel that their grief is being measured by the gestational age of their baby. We have known many examples of women who have had later losses who have been ready to go back to work before those whose baby died before 24 weeks' gestation. In cases like this, the support we offer women includes writing to employers to explain the nature of the individual's grief and advise their continued absence from work. Any return to work should be negotiated, with the mother taking the lead. A return to work succeeds best when it is staggered and within the control of the woman. A gradual resumption of duties will enable her to regain and retain control. She has to rebuild her mental and physical muscles just as if she had been off with a physical illness. This regaining of strength will certainly take weeks or, more probably, months.

REMEMBERING

Women worry that when their pain begins to lessen it means that they have stopped caring for their baby and they are frightened they are forgetting the baby. We try to reassure them that this is not the case; that they would need to have the part of their brain that deals with memory removed to forget their baby. Keeping the memory of their baby alive is essential and part of establishing a continuing bond. As a caregiver, you can help by including the baby in your ongoing dealings with mothers, fathers and their families. In any future pregnancy, you can mention the baby that died; you can talk about the next baby being a brother or sister of the deceased baby.

Mementoes and rituals are essential for helping to ensure continued acknowledgement of the baby's existence. Individuals find their own way of commemorating their beloved baby; some create a special corner in the garden, some light a candle weekly or yearly. One woman we know goes to church on the monthly anniversary of the date of the death of her daughter. You can help by talking to bereaved parents about the ways they have for the continued honouring of their baby. From my own personal experience, I (Sheila) am able to tell bereaved patients about the uncle of my brother-in-law who must have been born at the very beginning of the twentieth century and who died soon after his birth. I know him to have been called William. I know that every year on William's birthday his parents and their other children marked his day by having a special tea. This sense of love for William who did not survive has been passed down to the next generation and even to me, an in-law. As a way of helping them to know that their baby, too, can go on existing in the hearts and minds of others, I point out to them that here we are in the twenty-first century talking about William and recalling his existence.

SUMMARY

The death of a baby brings about intense anguish and pain. Sometimes this level of pain frightens women, their partners and families. They need support throughout the time they grieve. As one woman said recently, when she was worried that after 4 months of unrelenting grief she had stopped grieving, 'Is that all my pain amounts to, 4 months?' She realised quickly that her grief had not ended. This illustrates one of the contradictions of grief: that in the midst of it you want it to stop, and when it is absent, it feels as if something is missing.

REFERENCES

1. Encyclopedia of Death and Dying. *Continuing Bonds*. Encyclopedia of Death and Dying; n.d. Available at: www.deathreference.com/Ce-Da/Continuing-Bonds.html (accessed 23 August 2012).
2. Thomas J, Samuel J. Women, men and grief (Child Bereavement Charity information sheet). Available at: www.childbereavement.org.uk

CHAPTER 13

The next pregnancy

INTRODUCTION

Patients will want to talk about the next pregnancy at different times. Some will talk about it naturally; in other cases, the onus will be on the staff to start the conversation. Some women will ask almost straight away, even before their dead baby is delivered, about when they will be able to try for another pregnancy. For most, the grief of their current loss overwhelms their thoughts and they are not able to see past the next few hours, let alone as far as the next pregnancy. This gamut of responses means that you may find yourself talking to a woman about the next pregnancy whenever she asks questions about it, even if this seems to you to be unfeasibly soon or, alternatively, you may have to raise the subject tentatively, much later in the process.

For some women, the task of conceiving again may be fraught with difficulty. Some women may have had years of infertility investigations followed by failed attempts at IVF, and find themselves in their 40s with or perhaps without a partner. For them, the notion of trying again looks like an insurmountable hurdle and this should only be discussed by someone with experience and tact. Other women may get pregnant easily and they will be eager to talk about how to make sure they have a break before conceiving again.

Some discussions about the next pregnancy will be important from the perspective of patient safety; for example, if the woman has had serious problems related to hypertension, she will need to have her blood pressure effectively controlled before she conceives again. A senior clinician must embark on this conversation before the woman leaves hospital, in case this is the only opportunity to discuss the details.

Most maternity units will make arrangements to meet women and their partners following their pregnancy loss to discuss test results and to answer their questions. This will usually be about 6 to 8 weeks after the loss, by which time the results of tests including, hopefully, PM examination findings will be available. This may be a good time to raise the issue of future pregnancies if they are ready to have this conversation.

'WHEN CAN I GET PREGNANT AGAIN?'

There may be reasons why it might be a good idea for the patient to wait before embarking on the next pregnancy, but for some women the desire to try again quickly will be very strong indeed. There are many factors to consider before you can discuss this, including the woman's age, whether it was difficult for her to get pregnant in the first place, whether she needed infertility treatment, whether a similar loss has happened before and whether she has had previous pregnancy losses investigated. It is very important not to make assumptions about how easy it will be for her to get pregnant again, as for some the process will be complex and stressful.

Sometimes women will want to be pregnant again quite soon after the death of their baby and they feel guilty about this. They feel they are betraying the baby who died and not really caring about her. We deal with this by acknowledging their feelings and saying that it is all right to want another baby. They wanted the baby that died and the death of that baby does not take away the desire to have a live, healthy baby. Women may need reassurance that they can honour the memory of their baby that died and go on to have a brother or sister for that baby.

Talking about when to try again for another baby can cause anxiety for the staff and for the parents. A doctor may feel that she or he does not know how to approach the subject in the right manner, and the patient may feel too frightened to do so, perhaps fearing another disaster or that she will be told that another pregnancy would be too risky for her. This is especially so if the birth was traumatic and clinically complicated.

Some members of staff will suggest a time frame for trying again. Examples of such time frames are discussed below.

➤ *'You should wait for 3 months'.* This is often said because women will hopefully by then have had two normal periods, and if they were to conceive again they would be clear about the date of their last period and thus be confident about being able to date the pregnancy. There is no real medical justification for this, since, once a pregnancy test is positive, the woman would be able to have a scan to assess the gestation accurately. Furthermore, there is a drawback with this time frame because of the potential clashing of dates between the anniversary of the loss and the estimated date of delivery of the new pregnancy – if the woman conceives 3 months after her loss, the date of the last baby's death and the date of the new baby's birth may nearly or actually coincide.

➤ *'You should wait for a year'*. A woman will often be told to wait for a year, especially if her baby was delivered by a CS. The reason for saying this is not obvious and may be either because of emotional or surgical concerns. It may be because there is an increased risk of scar rupture if a woman attempts a VBAC within a year of having a CS, and the risk of scar rupture during a VBAC diminishes somewhat after a year. An instruction to wait for a year is almost always unnecessary, mainly because a woman whose baby died despite her having had a CS would be unlikely to choose to deliver by a VBAC next time. If the reason for the advice is emotional rather than surgical, the 1-year wait may be fine for some couples but an eternity for others. Staff often advise that women should wait a year, but it is not always clear what they mean. Do they mean that a woman should wait a year before conceiving or that she should aim to give birth again at least a year after the loss? Does waiting a year mean not trying to get pregnant again for 12 months or does it mean that it is safe to be pregnant again in a year's time? If it means the latter then when do they start to attempt to conceive? It could take one try or many more tries. Our suspicion is that staff give this advice because they feel it would be better if they say something, even if what they say does not have much (or any) evidence supporting it.

If you have found yourself falling into this trap, you need to be aware that patients may hang on to your advice more than you anticipate. Unless there are clear obstetric reasons for delaying, the discussion about the next pregnancy needs to include the mother's and father's concerns about timing and their fears and hopes of a successful outcome next time. If you give advice, it should be based on the mother's medical condition and the parents' concerns, rather than picking a random time frame simply because you want to say something.

➤ *'You should wait until you are both ready'*. On the surface, this may seem to be a good maxim, but it is not always easy, because the mother and father may feel ready at different times and in different ways. The woman's partner might be frightened about what could happen if she was to become pregnant again and then went on to suffer another loss, and may wish to protect her from any of that happening again. Alternatively, the woman may feel that she must try to become pregnant again as soon as possible, almost as if to verify that she is still really a woman. Of course, the couple may see the dilemma the other way round, with the mother frightened to try again and her partner desperate to feel that he can be a father without any delay.

The appearance of her period each month will serve as a reminder for the woman that she is not pregnant and she may feel as if she has wasted another month. The last time she had periods was before she conceived the baby who died, and it can be difficult for her to have her body resume its biological functioning so easily whilst her emotional being is still in so much pain.

MEDICAL CONSIDERATIONS BEFORE ANOTHER PREGNANCY

There may be important medical reasons why a woman should wait before trying to conceive again. She may have a condition that needs to be correctly stabilised prior to another pregnancy, such as hypertension or diabetes. Conceiving again before any such condition is controlled would be unsafe for her and increase her risk of having a further pregnancy loss. The woman may need to see another specialist before becoming pregnant again, such as a neurologist if she is an epileptic on anticonvulsants or a cardiologist if she has heart problems. You can assist her by arranging the necessary appointments or organising a referral.

   You will also need to give the patient advice about medication once she starts trying to conceive. She needs to know when she should start taking any medication before becoming pregnant (such as folic acid) and when she should stop any (such as tetracyclines for acne).

PLANS FOR THE NEXT PREGNANCY

We have found that whatever the circumstances or gestation of the previous loss, women are keen or, more correctly, anxious to have some professional contact early in the next pregnancy, so that they can be reassured that the pregnancy has started well. This is understandable in someone with a history of recurrent first trimester loss, and there is evidence to support the use of early scans and reassurance for these women as a way of improving pregnancy outcome,[1] but most bereaved women benefit from early pregnancy support. Any plan for care during a future pregnancy must include appropriate contact details, so that women can make direct and definite arrangements to be seen early in their next pregnancy by someone who knows their history. A woman's GP may well be able to arrange an early appointment for her, and ensure that she has an early scan, but we have found that women's experiences of negotiating this can sometimes be patchy and uncertain. We prefer that women make direct contact themselves without any potential hurdles to jump. This will usually be by telephone or email, and include the option of contacting the counsellors' office as well as the doctor or midwife.

When discussing the timing of another pregnancy, we have found it helpful to assure a couple that they will be able to contact one or both of us when they are pregnant again and that their care will start from that point. They need to be able to discuss the details of what will happen, including early scans and appointments, and the arranging of blood tests and any other relevant medical care. Moreover, they need be able to access emotional support that may, if necessary, continue throughout the next pregnancy. The details of these arrangements are written in a letter to the parents after they have been discussed, so that they have written confirmation about the plan when they are pregnant again. The letter is copied to the GP so that he or she is also aware of these details. It is very important that the patient has her own copy of this letter, with a detailed plan about how she should be cared for in a future pregnancy, so that she does not have to remember everything that she has been told. With the help of her letter, she will be able to state clearly what she needs, in case any of her future caregivers are not sure. This is vital if she is being looked after at a different hospital from where she had the previous loss. This might be out of necessity, if the couple move house, for example, or might be by choice, because they cannot bear the thought of returning to the hospital where their baby died. A copy of this letter will be filed in the patient's hospital notes. In our experience, these are not always available for a community midwife doing a booking appointment, which makes it all the more necessary to give a copy of the letter to the patient, so that she can show it to her midwife.

THE NEXT PREGNANCY

Whether it is weeks, months or years after the death of their baby, it is likely that the woman and her partner will be scared once they know that she is pregnant again. If she wishes to return to the same hospital, you will hear from her because of what you said and confirmed in the letter following their loss. It is imperative, as we have emphasised throughout this book, that her care is patient-centred. In our dealings with women who have had the experience of a pregnancy loss, what they want is to be looked after by as few people as possible. They need and want consistent, dependable care from their GP, an experienced midwife and senior doctor. They do not want to have to be repeating their previous experience or explaining why they feel like they do to new people all the time. They may want to be looked after by the same people who were involved during the last pregnancy and with the death of their baby, or they may want to have completely different people.

Just as it is good practice not to make assumptions when you are working with a woman at the time of the death of her baby, you should not pre-judge how she is managing during the next pregnancy. For example, we know one woman, who was childless, who had two ectopic pregnancies. She could never imagine that she would have a successful pregnancy and a live baby, but she got pregnant again. Initially, she was terrified that history would repeat itself and, when it did not, she found it difficult to be in unfamiliar territory. She knew much better how to deal with a pregnancy ending than she did with it continuing. This is a fairly common type of reaction and you need to understand the different dilemmas that women face during their next pregnancy. We set up support for her: she had access to one specialist midwife, a counsellor and a consultant obstetrician. The consultant was also the person who had looked after her when she had had her ectopic pregnancies and therefore someone in whom she had faith. When she was 20 weeks' pregnant, she saw another doctor at her appointment, the consultant being absent, and this doctor told her that she did not really need to be attending this clinic any more, as she was now considered low risk and that as doctors, they could not really tell her anything different from a midwife. Whilst it was true that, in the strictest sense of the word, she was not having a 'difficult' pregnancy, her history and her personality made it impossible for her to be treated in the same way as any other patient who had not experienced a loss. This situation was quickly put right by the other people caring for her and she continued to see the consultant. This was not because her pregnancy was threatened but because she needed to be treated with 'tender loving care' and because of the faith she had in the doctor. This was psychologically hugely important to her. If the woman had come to her own conclusion that she no longer needed to attend the consultant's clinic, this would have been a completely different matter.

Working with the anxieties of women, their partners and sometimes their wider families regarding the next pregnancy is challenging but hugely worthwhile. We expect that women will be anxious and we will tell them in advance of them getting pregnant that it is part of our job to support them with their worries. We cannot guarantee them a baby at the end but we can accompany them during the weeks and months of their pregnancy. They know they will be cared for.

One particular anxiety relates to the labour ward itself. If the last time a woman was on the labour ward was when her baby died, it is little wonder that she will be frightened by the thought of going there again. It can be helpful for her to visit the labour ward with someone who understands what she has been through, before she is admitted to have her baby, so that she can defuse some of her anxieties. This also gives the opportunity for any feelings that arise to be expressed and explored. In this way, these feelings can be separated from the anticipation of the new baby. One example of this concerns a woman whose baby had died following a difficult instrumental delivery. Her next baby was to be delivered by a planned CS, but she was frightened by the thought of going back into the operating theatre. She found it extremely helpful to visit the labour ward, and the operating theatre in particular, in advance of her admission. During the visit, she was tearful and upset, which was to be expected, but it meant that she was not overwhelmed by these feelings when she came in to have her new baby.

Women worry that their anxiety will have a negative effect on the baby, but it is asking the impossible to expect that someone who has had a pregnancy loss will be able to be anxiety-free in a future pregnancy. Giving women permission to be anxious can free them from at least berating themselves for being scared. Many women do not stop being nervous or apprehensive until there is a baby in their arms.

It is worth remembering, too, that it is pointless telling patients not to worry. If they had that much control over their worries that they could stop, then they would not be worried in the first place. It can helpful to know that it is not your job to stop a woman and her family worrying, as you will not be able to do so. You need to listen to her worries and, if there are practical things that you can do or say which can counteract her concerns, then it is all right to give her that information. For example, if she is worried she will have to wait for her expected due date and is terrified of her baby dying during labour, you can discuss with her the merits of not waiting until then and talk with her about ways of delivering the baby safely before her due date. This information will not necessarily stop her worrying, but at least you are addressing her concerns. You need to know that if you have reassured her about having more control about the delivery date and method, as soon as that anxiety goes, another will pop up. This is the nature of anxiety and many women are scared not to be anxious; they do not feel safe taking things for granted, as they feel that if they do and something goes wrong again, they will be at fault for being careless enough not to worry.

Additionally, some women will try not to get too attached to the baby they are carrying. They are trying to avoid being so hurt again in the case of something going wrong with this pregnancy, too. Again, you need to be non-judgemental about this way of coping and know in reality that they are attached but cannot bring themselves to feel consciously that they are.

SUMMARY

Before another pregnancy, women need to have any medical problems addressed and to have contact details, so that they can alert their consultant or midwife when they know that they are pregnant again. From then on, as the doctor or midwife, you must do exactly what you have said you would do. Women will need emotional as well as medical support and this must be planned and organised with the same attention to detail as clinic appointments and scans have been. Special attention needs to be paid to particular dates, especially the anniversary of the last loss or of the last due date, and to particular gestations. A woman will be especially anxious when the gestation of her new pregnancy coincides with that of her previous loss. These times are significant and she may well benefit from being seen more frequently for reassurance at these times. Providing supportive care in this way can be very time-consuming and demanding but is profoundly rewarding.

REFERENCE

1. Clifford K, Rai R, Regan L. Future pregnancy outcome in unexplained recurrent first trimester miscarriage. *Hum Reprod.* 1997; **12**(2): 387–9.

CHAPTER 14

Training

INTRODUCTION

This chapter looks at some of what staff require to be able to do pregnancy-loss work and how their skills might be enhanced through training. We give examples of exercises that you can use to improve your understanding of and empathy with bereaved parents. We have also included some of the issues that arise in the training exercises. There are bound to be more, and you may come up with your own, but here are some starting points.

We have said previously that there is a debate to be had as to whether only those with a natural ability to care for bereaved parents should be doing it. Whatever hospitals and other institutions decide, all those involved in looking after women, their dead babies and their families need training and deserve to have support to provide the best care possible. Training comes in many forms and organisations such as Sands, the Miscarriage Association and the Child Bereavement Charity provide bereavement-related learning opportunities. The first two agencies will provide training within hospitals and other venues and it is possible to plan training that is specifically geared to your needs. Alternatively, you can, if you have experienced staff, provide your own training; we have provided pregnancy-loss training over the years. In this way we have been able to tailor the learning to the needs of individual staff and to reflect the diverse needs of staff and the patient population in our area. In a nutshell, what staff need to learn is how to care for bereaved parents, deal with the death of a baby and how their own fears and prejudices might interfere with good care. They need to have a chance to examine these fears and prejudices and practise alternative and better ways of providing care. This will almost certainly involve examining communication and how to communicate better, including giving bad news.

Initial training needs to help us look at our own attitudes to death and grief; to enable us to understand where we find it hard to cope and where we find it easier to manage. Being able to explore the 'places' that we find difficult within ourselves will make it less likely that we will want to avoid these areas with patients. For example, if you cannot cope with someone's distress at having had a number of miscarriages, and despair about whether they will ever have a baby, you might tell them 'at least you can get pregnant' in an attempt to encourage them. We know women who have had this said to them. A much more appropriate response would be to acknowledge how hopeless and helpless she is feeling. If we find our own hopelessness or feelings of not having control challenging, we will want to stop a patient expressing her painful emotions. We need to learn how not to do this.

People often find it difficult to witness anger or to be on the receiving end of it. However, the more you understand your own anger, the less likely you are to want to stop someone expressing their pain in this manner. Training can help you to explore this in a protected way.

Earlier, we mentioned that patients are sometimes criticised behind their backs and this is usually because they are behaving in a fashion or expressing emotions that particular staff members cannot deal with. For example, if patients are assertive they may be labelled a nuisance. This will make the staff member feel better. If patients behave in a manner that is outside of the staff members' understanding and is uncomfortable, it is likely that the patient will be seen as difficult. In fact, the patient's behaviour may be understandable because they are grieving, but the staff find it hard to cope with. An example of this would be calling for hospital security if a bereaved father is shouting and swearing on being told of his baby's death. Criticising patients and their relatives in this manner is a defence mechanism and training can help us to become aware of how this can interfere with caring. It can also provide us with alternative and better coping strategies.

No one really wants to give bad news because it would be better if there were no bad news to give. However, we believe that if staff are given the right training regarding 'giving bad news' then this task can be seen as an opportunity to be the best human being you can in the face of difficult or even unbearable events. So instead of metaphorically going to the back of the queue, hoping someone else will step forward, you would feel confident in your ability to take on the task of telling parents that their baby has died. What is difficult is the fact of the baby's death, not that we have to tell them. We are not suggesting it is easy by any means, but it is important to separate out the fact from the task.

Role play as a training technique

We have found that many people do not like role play and will avoid participating if they can. We think this is a shame, as it is an opportunity to experience what each player in the scenario of a baby's death may feel. It may be more useful to think about it as an opportunity to learn and develop your empathy for patients and to increase your confidence as a practitioner. Learning like this is demanding but then so is the real work. Learning through role play means your ego needs to get out of the way.

When doing role play, it is important to pay attention to your feelings, emotions, thoughts and physical reactions to whichever role you are in. Try not to focus too much on being good at being the patient, midwife or doctor; rather, see if you can get a sense of what it is like to be that person. Working through feeling embarrassed about your acting skills is nothing compared with causing pain and hurt to patients by saying the wrong thing. If you get hung up and embarrassed about whether your acting is up to scratch then it could be that you will assign these feelings of embarrassment to being in the role rather than what it feels like to be involved in a baby's death. Include your embarrassment and then explore how relevant it was to the scenario you were enacting, rather than just you not wanting to make a fool of yourself. For example, many women regard themselves as being sophisticated, assertive females but get annoyed and embarrassed with themselves when they are tongue-tied, nervous or anxious in a medical setting.

It is useful to note what you learnt about yourself in a particular role, what you learnt about others from them being in their roles and then to give each other feedback about what did and did not help. It is important to remember that when giving feedback you need to include positive aspects as well as saying what was not helpful. People will find different aspects of the scenarios easier or harder to deal with, and learning from each other can be of enormous help.

We all need to be humble enough to understand what mothers, fathers and others feel when a baby dies. This does not make us unprofessional; rather, it makes us better caregivers. Learning by making mistakes (and making mistakes is one of the best ways of learning) with our peers and colleagues can be very creative and illuminating.

Professional actors are extremely useful when role playing patients. They can bring their expertise to the task and make the encounter very realistic – maybe shockingly so. With an appropriate script, based on a real case or an amalgam of similar cases, actors can bring the scene to life and help those taking part to understand how patients might feel. Later in the day, or on another occasion, staff can role play patients and combine what they know from their professional experience and what they have learnt from watching the actors.

Whilst some members of staff might feel embarrassed about taking part in any role-play exercises, they should at least role play staff. They can bring their own experiences to the situation they are asked to enact then try to role play other members of staff, perhaps someone they have witnessed managing a situation well, whom they feel they could try to copy. They might also want to try role playing a staff member whom they have witnessed dealing badly with a situation and gauge the reaction of the group to this.

IDEAS FOR ROLE PLAY

As a result of our experience, we have come up with the following scenarios. We explore some of the feelings that might be engendered in those who take part and have suggested some ideas on which to reflect. In the scenarios, we have suggested that the staff member is either a doctor or a midwife, but, in most cases, these will be interchangeable.

➤ Try role playing the patient whilst someone else plays the doctor, explaining that you have an IUFD. Try doing this whilst lying on a bed or trolley with your colleague standing at the end of the bed/standing alongside you/sitting down next to you. Swap roles.

In this exercise, if you are role playing the doctor, you not only have the task of deciding on the words you will use when talking to the patient, but you also have to make decisions about your posture and physical stance. Your body language will betray how you are feeling both personally and professionally. It may seem normal to stand over a patient, and there is some comfort for you in feeling normal, but the dynamics of the encounter are very different if you are alongside the patient at the same level. It is interesting to use the same script with the 'doctor' in a different position each time and to assess how that feels for both people taking part. Which felt best for the doctor? Which felt best for the patient?

➤ Role play being the midwife or doctor whilst another colleague is the patient or employ actors to do this. Try explaining to them what happens during an induction of labour for a dead baby whilst they stay completely silent. Then try doing the same thing but with the person role playing the patient constantly weeping.

People staying silent can be very disconcerting, as you will not get verbal cues from them. Instead, in this scenario, you need to try to notice what their body language was telling you. Did they look at you? If not, where was their focus? Who was with them or were they on they own? If so, did you check if they wanted someone close to be there before beginning? Did you suggest that they may need someone else there to take in what is being said?

Someone weeping can be disconcerting too. Did you acknowledge how upsetting the news was that you were giving them? Did you check if they wanted some time to themselves before you continued or whether you could carry on even if they were upset? Did you find their distress frightening?

➤ Try discussing consent for a PM whilst the patient continually asks questions and keeps interrupting.

This is interesting because it mimics the way that some patients behave. They will be so desperate for answers that they will rush on to the next question before they have really taken in the response to the previous one. Their brains are running too fast for their thoughts, and they race from one question to the next without time to let anything sink in. If you are role playing the doctor in this situation, one tactic is simply to stop talking whenever the patient butts in, and calmly go back to the beginning of whatever it was that was being said, in an effort to finish the point that you were trying to make. This can be very frustrating because you want to try to finish what you are saying and move on, but it is a useful exercise to learn to be patient in a situation like this. As the doctor, you have your script (the PM consent form) and you want to move logically from one section to the next, but patients do not know the script and will often have lots of questions about each point. As well as this, they may be particularly concerned about one point, which may seem inconsequential to you, but which matters a great deal to them and thus you must give your full attention to this.

Another tactic would be to acknowledge that the patient has a lot of questions and that to answer them will take longer than perhaps they had anticipated. It would be acceptable to ask them to slow down in order to help you to address all of their queries and, if time is short, suggest that you will return later on to continue the discussion.

➤ Practise discussing the results of a PM with a patient and her partner
   when there is a congenital abnormality. Practise doing the same thing
   when there is no abnormality.

These two discussions can feel very different. There may be a certain
relief in having to talk about an abnormality, since it means that there
is an explanation for the pregnancy loss. There might be structural
abnormalities, genetic problems or a syndrome of some kind on
which to hang your professional hat. You are in a horrible situation,
but at least you have something to talk about. In contrast, when there
is no abnormality and, perhaps, therefore, no explanation for what
went wrong, the way that you talk will be different and may almost be
apologetic. Sometimes a normal result will be expected, for example,
if the baby has died because of a massive placental abruption, and the
patient may be relieved that there was nothing else wrong. For many,
though, the news that there was no abnormality will open the door to
even more questions – 'Well, what was it then?' – to which you do not
have the answers. It is useful to rehearse what you would say in this
situation, so that you can produce a form of words that is clear and
sympathetic, whilst at the same time acknowledging that this 'normal'
news is difficult to hear.

Try doing each with different seating arrangements: for example, with
you sitting side by side with the couple or sitting opposite. You may find
that sitting side by side makes it easier to discuss a complex report, as you
will be able to show them sections of it and perhaps draw diagrams to
explain any structural abnormality. When you sit opposite a patient, you
may feel 'protected', but you might seem distant and superior to them.
With a number of people to include, say, in a small family group, you
could try sitting in a circle and see if this feels better.

What was the difference between telling people that their baby
had a congenital abnormality and telling them that there was no such
problem? Was the former easier because there was an actual reason for
the death? Did you resort to using the medical terminology used in the
PM report or did you use non-medical language?

➤ Practise saying something to the patient and then being silent to let it
   sink in. Stay silent for a full minute to see how it feels. Practise *not* filling
   the silences. Try role playing a patient being silent.

After telling someone momentous information, it may be necessary
for you to give time to let it sink in. You can let people know that you are

going to give them a minute or two to take the news in and for them to formulate any questions. Do not absent yourself physically or mentally at this point, but stay alert to the nuances of what is going on with the patient and any companions.

Silence is sometimes one of the most difficult responses to deal with, as there are few clues to tell you how you are doing or how what you are saying is being received. If patients are silent, it may be important to stay silent yourself for a little while. You can ask them if they want you to be silent with them. If you are getting uncomfortable with that or sense that the patient is unsure about what you are doing, say that you are just being there and that if they want you they just need to talk to you. Alternatively, you can ask them if they would prefer to be on their own, in which case you will come back and see them later. If you do this, you need to be careful that you are not giving them the message that you just want to be out of the room as quickly as possible.

➤ Role play an angry patient who thinks a midwife did something wrong that resulted in her baby dying. Have someone else role play the senior midwife or doctor who explains what happened and acknowledges that a mistake was made. Then do the same thing but this time with the senior person explaining that no one made a mistake; that is, that her baby died for other reasons and that it was no one's fault.

In the first place, you need to acknowledge the person's anger without being defensive or sounding too formulaic. You can say that you understand that she is angry and agree that, unfortunately, she has good reason for her anger. It really helps the patient if, as the senior person, you say that what she thinks is correct and that a mistake was actually made for which you apologise. This is very powerful because patients will usually expect staff to try to cover up any mistakes made by their colleagues.

What happened to the patient's demeanour when the fault was acknowledged? Were you then able to have a discussion in which she could take in what was being said and speak about her own experience without her anger getting in the way? Did you suggest to the patient how she might proceed with a formal complaint now that she has heard your explanation? How did that feel? Did you feel as though you were betraying your colleague or did you feel empowered to help the patient because you were being open and honest? Did the prospect of causing a problem for the hospital worry you?

If you were role playing the angry patient, what was it like to have your feelings acknowledged? Did the acknowledgment feel authentic? What was it like when the senior clinician agreed with you?

In the second version, you will need to explore with the patient, in a non-defensive way, why she thinks that the midwife made a mistake. You need to listen with an open mind initially and not jump in to defend your colleague. It may be that the patient feels that a perceived lack of care correlates with her baby's death; in other words, if only the midwife had cared for her in an appropriate way then she believes her baby would have survived. It is important to acknowledge her reality whilst remaining clear that no actual mistakes were made. The potential pitfall here is that in explaining that it was no one's fault, you can make it sound like something is being covered up or that a rogue colleague is being protected. The patient is desperate for an answer and you have not provided one that makes any sense to her, so she may continue to believe her own version of events rather than yours. You may just have to accept this. How does this make you feel? Have you lost sympathy for the patient or are you still able to be empathic? How do you feel about your colleague in the light of the patient alleging that she did not care for her appropriately? Were you able to acknowledge that, whilst no actual mistake was responsible for the death of her baby, she may have a complaint to make with regard to her care?

➤ Practise saying 'I'm sorry this has happened' and 'I'm sorry for your loss'. This is different from saying 'I'm sorry that I let you down' or 'I'm sorry I made a mistake'.

This is different from the previous scenario. This is about conveying to the patient and her family that you have some idea about the enormity of their loss. Many members of staff will have been told in the past not to apologise to patients when something goes wrong, for fear of admitting liability. It is now recognised that saying sorry is a profoundly important thing to do that will be appreciated and remembered by patients.

➤ Role play a midwife or doctor who has been asked by a bereaved father to tell his children that the baby has gone to heaven to be with the other angels. Have someone role play the children.

Did you find this easy? If so, what made it easy? Did it matter that you may not share his beliefs? If you thought it inappropriate to fulfil the father's request, how did you manage the situation? Did you suggest that you could help him tell his children what he wanted them to know?

There is no right or wrong here; it will be down to your own individual preferences. It is worth practising being asked to do things out of the ordinary and find out how you respond. Give yourself time to find out what you are in fact being asked to do (remember the statement behind the question) and time to decide how you respond.

➤ The patient talks to you (as a midwife or doctor) about wanting to carry her baby son in her arms on the way to his funeral. She has been told by someone else that she will make things worse for herself if she does this.

In this scenario, you need to explain to her that there is no right or wrong in this situation and help her by exploring what 'making things worse' means to her. It can be helpful to use your hands to help her weigh up the situation: on one hand, find out what is important to her about carrying her son in her arms; on the other, find out if she actually has any objections to doing this or is it that someone has planted a doubt in her mind? This way she may be able to come to the best decision she can for herself.

OTHER HELPFUL TRAINING EXERCISES

➤ If you are confident about handling a dead baby, encourage your junior colleagues and students to practise seeing and holding them. Help them to get used to how it feels to do this without becoming disrespectful.

If we are to help bereaved parents see and hold their dead babies, we need to be confident about doing this ourselves, however strange and unsettling it may initially feel. Sometimes a dead baby will be placed in a room away from the parents before being taken to the mortuary, and this provides a good opportunity for a senior staff member to involve a junior colleague or a student. This is partly so that they can see that holding the baby is not frightening or difficult and that the baby's body is not going to break, and partly to show that handling the baby is a normal thing to do. It can be serious without necessarily being solemn.

➤ Think of words that mean one thing to medical personnel and another to everyone else, for example, 'tissue', 'products', and try to construct sentences using different words instead.

Additionally, you could come up with ways that these words are used in everyday speech, as this will help you to understand how they are perceived by patients.

Alternative words for 'tissue' could include 'flesh', 'skin', 'muscle', 'nerve', or 'pieces of' liver, kidney and so on. Alternative terms for 'products' could be 'the remainder of the pregnancy', 'the remains of the pregnancy', 'what is left of the pregnancy', 'the rest of the pregnancy'.

Here are some examples:

> 'The pathologist will take tiny samples/slivers/pieces of your baby's liver to examine under a microscope.' You need to be as explicit as you can be about the size of the sample, as 'tiny' to you may not mean the same as it does to someone else.

> 'You will need to have a surgical procedure to remove what is left of the pregnancy from your womb; this is so that there is no danger of you developing an infection.'

> 'You need a surgical procedure to empty your womb of the pregnancy.'

> 'You need to have a procedure to empty your womb.'

> 'The people in the laboratory will look carefully at what is removed from your womb to see if they can explain what went wrong with your pregnancy.'

Help each other out by suggesting different responses and practise them on each other.

➤ Think of the last time you could not find your keys or you lost your purse or wallet and this will call to mind feelings of helplessness, blame of self or others, confusion, lack of control, anger, frustration and sadness about not being able to recover the object. These are just some of the states that begin to describe grief and bereavement. By having some idea of these you will have an impression of what mothers and fathers go through when their babies die.

SUMMARY

Initial and ongoing training is vital if staff are to have the knowledge and understanding of the emotional, mental and practical aspects of care involved in looking after bereaved parents. An adequate structure can be in place for the completion of practical tasks, for example, with a checklist, but if staff do not understand the nuances involved, mistakes are likely to happen. For example, we recently saw a commemorative certificate with 'male infant' instead of the baby's given name and surname. This showed that the midwife had no idea of the significance of the certificate. It would have been very inappropriate and detrimental to have given it to the bereaved mother. The checklist might say 'give the mother a commemorative certificate', but, without insight or train-ing, the midwife merely ticked the box without understanding the importance of naming the baby. In this instance, it is fortunate that the mother was given a card with her baby's name and the significance of her loss was recognised appropriately.

We hope that with training, staff will become more confident in their ability. This means that bereaved parents and their families will receive the treatment they require and hospital trusts will probably benefit from having fewer complaints. Supporting each other through the process of learning will better equip you to do this challenging work and enable you to provide the best care you can for your patients.

Index